The
Sugar Detox Solution

A Beginner's Guide To Eliminate Cravings and
Overcome Sugar Addiction

by

Monica E. Harris

Your Free Gift

Thank you for choosing this book on how to complete a sugar detox!

As a special thank you, I would love to send you a collection of Printable Planners as a FREE gift.

This 4 sheet set of PDFs includes printables of the following:

- 7 Day Sugar Detox Meal Plan
- Sugar Free Desserts and Snacks Recipes
- A Sugar Detox Shopping List
- A Weekly Food Diary

Each sheet was designed to make it easier to start your sugar detox journey.

Simply go to the following URL to claim your **FREE** gift:

https://tinyurl.com/SugarDetoxFreebies

Disclaimer

The Sugar Detox Solution
First edition. January 22, 2021.
Copyright © 2021 Monica E. Harris

Table of Contents

Introduction

It's no secret that sugar can be hard to resist. In today's world, people are regularly consuming unhealthy amounts of added sugar daily, which is directly linked to increased cases of obesity, diabetes and heart-related diseases. Once you are hooked by irresistible cravings, breaking free may feel like an impossible task. The love for sugar might seem harmless at first, but studies have shown that we are consuming much more than we need.

According to research conducted by New Harvard School Of Public Health, over 180,000 people die globally every year as a result of sweetened-beverage consumption. Of this alarming figure, the United States alone accounts for 25,000 deaths, which amounts to a staggering 14 percent. If you have decided to track your sugar intake, the task is made even more difficult since most nutrition labels tag sugar under unfamiliar names.

Even though soft drinks, pies, baked food, sweetened dairy, and candy are some of the most popular sources of added sugar, it might be surprising to note that seemingly healthy foods like baked beans, bread, protein bars, and premade soup also contain unhealthy amounts of sugar. The natural source makes it easy to unknowingly consume their sugar content excessively.

Why Is Sugar Addiction So Hard To Beat?

While it is true that your health is uniquely your responsibility, it does not change the fact that we are always under the manipulation of big food companies. Over the years, they have worked tirelessly to alter our perception in making us believe that their chemical-ridden and factory-processed products are wholesome food for consumption. The qualifier 'organic' now needs to be added to natural, earth-harvested food to distinguish it from the junk we have been primed to eat daily. It is the biggest fraud of the century, and the foundation of this deception is as old as the advertisement industry that drives it.

Over the past 100 years, the quality of the food that we eat has progressively declined. It has become just one piece in an elaborate marketing ploy that includes peddling addictive substances to the public through effective advertising. An average dinner table at Thanksgiving now consists of more junk food and so-called "pre-made" meals than actual healthy, organic food. These sugary foods are mostly filled with sweeteners that initiate biochemical reactions in our bodies and cause our brains to become addicted to them. Another factor in this sugar epidemic is the unbridled access we currently have to these addictive substances. Addictive sugar products are simply everywhere. They have been strategically made to be cheaper, and more readily accessible, than organic food.

Unhealthy sugary foods also masquerade as a rewards system to gratify our addictions and keep us hooked. The phenomenon of 'comfort food' is an epidemic all unto itself. You might be feeling down or depressed and find yourself resorting to junk food to feel better. This is by no means an accident. This is called 'Food Addiction,' and its root can be traced to the effects excess sugar has on our body. Aside from the fact that sugar tastes really good, the reason that it is so hard to cut out is that refined sugar found in foods such as ice cream, cake, bread, and candy triggers your neurological rewards system. When you eat sugar, your brain's opioid activators kick into gear. Cutting out refined sugar from your diet causes your body to go into withdrawal, and you experience symptoms such as mood swings, headaches, cravings, reduced energy levels, and even hormonal imbalances in some cases.

Despite the negative physical effects of sugar, it still makes you feel good emotionally. When you deprive yourself of sugar, your body experiences a decrease in dopamine release. Dopamine is a neurotransmitter responsible for reward-motivated behavior and pleasure. What this means is that dopamine sends chemical signals to your brain, giving you the feeling of happiness when you consume sugar.

The Dangerous Grip of Sugar

It has been proven that sugar produces the same reaction an addictive drug would on the brain. Any attempt at quitting could kick in withdrawal symptoms such as headaches, muscle aches, fatigue, and even depression. When we consume sugary products, the hormones serotonin and endorphin are produced, which are known to create the feeling of happiness. After consuming sugary food, we are then left with a feeling of fleeting satisfaction and our brain makes an immediate chemical connection it. When you are down or having a bad day, your brain will try to 'solve' your mood by nudging you towards whatever food you consumed earlier that made you feel 'good'. This attempt by your brain to recapture that positive feeling traps you in a vicious cycle where you find yourself returning to a product that might damage your health.

All this information might seem bleak and make you feel powerless. The mass marketed food we eat on a daily basis affects us negatively, disrupting our productivity and taking away from our health. You may be wondering if you even have a chance at beating the addiction and leading a healthy lifestyle.

Rest assured, you can.

This book will tackle every part of how to break a sugar addiction, stop the endless cravings, and eventually lose weight.

In the next chapter, I will discuss the sugar epidemic in America and its consequences. I will also talk about the basic characteristics of sugar addiction, relevant scenarios, and relatable pointers that will help you notice it in yourself, your diet, and your loved ones' habits. After this, we will go in-depth into the national problem of sugar addiction and how society is currently endorsing it before showing the health implications this has for us. I will discuss the symptoms and present you with 5 key identifiers to quickly determine whether or not you have a true sugar addiction.

Not all sugar is harmful, however, and so chapter 2 will be dedicated to understanding the differences between good and bad sugar. I will explain how sugar can be healthy and unhealthy, and identify what type is beneficial to consume. We will also properly tackle the topic of added sugar, what it is and how to identify it. You will learn how it is detrimental to your health and how it eventually leads to addiction. You will also be provided with a quick guide on how to identify food with high sugar content.

In Chapter 3, you will discover the first recognizable steps towards your freedom from sugar addiction. We will dive into the topic of Sugar Detox and discuss the complete health benefits of detoxing your body. You will learn to identify the foods you should be eating and their health benefits. We will then focus on the much-needed topic of altering your eating habits and patterns and how to select specific foods that will help detox your system from sugar. You will be presented with detailed food ideas for Sugar Detox Meals, which will be clearly segmented into breakfast, dinner, lunch, and snack categories. I will also provide a 5 day and 7 day sugar detox meal plan.

In chapter 4, we will take a more fitness-oriented approach to eliminate sugar from the body. First, I will discuss how the body reacts to a sugar detox and how physical fitness can help you reach better results. Then I will outline a list of exercises that you can do while you are on your sugar detox diet. They will be divided into time categories ranging from 15-minute workout sessions to 90-minute workout sessions, while also giving you useful tips for exercises that you can fit into a busy schedule.

After discussing the nuances of achieving your desired results, we will deal with the task of maintaining these results in chapter 5. First, I will cover how to manage withdrawal syndromes associated with sugar cravings and how to practice daily mindfulness to help you cope. I will also provide food substitutions to help you stay faithful to your detox. Finally, we will conclude with the 'how' and 'why' of getting a support group for your newfound lifestyle.

My Story

The struggle with sugar addiction is one I personally identify with. Years of unhealthy eating habits that included heavy consumption of sugary foods left me overweight and living with spiked cholesterol levels. I also suffered from abnormal sleeping patterns as a result. I was depressed, emotionally imbalanced, and in desperate need of a change. It wasn't long before I was forced to recognize my own self-destructive routines.

I struggled with the negative effects of a high sugar diet until a lifelong friend, who was also a dietician, confronted me. Through her, I became aware of my eating habits and how they contributed to my health issues. I wanted to cut down the addiction so that I could achieve some relief and lead the life that I have always wanted—to be productive, healthy, and driven.

The steps she revealed to me helped drastically change the course of my eating habits and patterns. It wasn't easy at first. I resisted, relapsed and even considered ending our friendship. But as I pushed through, the results were life changing. After six months, I had lost 50 pounds of weight and lowered my cholesterol levels dramatically. My sleeping pattern also improved, and my overall well-being took a healthier turn. I found that I could now perform activities and do things that I previously only dreamt of doing. I found a new confidence, determination, and power in the new life I decided to adopt.

My personal transformation has placed me on a trajectory that seeks to see change in the world around me. I want people to be healthy, and all of my life choices have led me to this point. As you continue with me, I will show you exactly how to properly detox your body from the overconsumption of sugar and maintain choices proven to boost overall health.

We have heard the saying, *'nothing good comes easy'* a million times. At first, the steps in this book may be difficult to adopt, but this is also true about any new habit. Your brain and body will strike back, complain, and fight you. There will be days when you will feel like giving up, but you won't. The reason I know you won't is because you will have your eyes set on a prize-- the prize of a healthier lifestyle.

This book is a practical approach to cutting down your high sugar diet and detoxing your system. It is geared towards achieving a healthy and better standard of living. It is written as a 'manual' that will teach you how to fight and wage war on your body's natural tendency to choose the easier path of a high sugar diet. It is a step-by-step guide towards maintaining a healthier lifestyle and staying consistent with the healthy choices you will adopt.

The media attempts to mold us into mindless consumers, eating and reflecting the unhealthy choices they project. While sugar consumption is necessary if we want to function properly on a social and physiological level, it does not have to be mindless. We must not give in to the daily routine of unhealthy habits. We must take charge of our lives and live consciously, aware of what we consume daily, whether it is eating with others or by ourselves.

I want to personally thank you for choosing this book. There is no better time than now to win the battle against sugar addiction.

Let's get started together on the journey to a healthier you!

1. THE SUGAR EPIDEMIC AND ITS CONSEQUENCES

It seems as if sugar is nearly impossible to avoid. From frosted cookies to sweetened yogurts and strawberry cupcakes, sugar is everywhere. We have been primed both emotionally and psychologically to depend on these sugary substances. Whether we like it or not, these foods create surplus sugar in our body once ingested. To put the gravity of our situation into perspective, studies have revealed that a staggering 75% of Americans today eat more sugar than their body needs. Ignorance is certainly not bliss when it comes to your health. What you do not know *can* harm you, and that is why I have dedicated the first chapter to the following topics:

1. Outlining the characteristics and symptoms of sugar addiction so you will know exactly what to look for.
2. Discussing the larger problem of society and its role in contributing to the high sugar content problem in America.
3. Breaking down exactly how a high sugar diet can damage your health and affect your general well-being.

Characteristics Of A Sugar Addiction

Sugar addiction is a lot easier to spot when compared to other substance-based addictions. When taking an objective approach, 5 unique behavioral disorders can be identified as telltale signs of a sugar addiction. These identifiers are based on measuring how a person consumes their food or drinks.

1. Emotional Eating

In a sad or uncomfortable situation, anything that brings the slightest trace of relief is welcome. It's not surprising that people will resort to the sweet taste of sugar in moments of weakness, irritation, or grief. One of the effects of sugar in our bodies is the instant energy it provides, which serves as a 'quick fix' for anyone who wants to forge through their long days. For example, Hollywood's portrayal of what comes immediately after a break-up is not too far from the truth. I would argue that it is actually spot on. This involves television, a tub of ice cream and a couch, serving as the temporary distraction from the grief and heartache people suffer.

The flip side to this is most, if not all, get addicted to the sugary substance. They become dependent on the temporary relief that tub of sugar provides. This often distracts them from doing other important things in their lives, which ultimately leads to weight gain, a feeling of helplessness, and damage to the individual's self-esteem. As mentioned earlier, it is a vicious cycle that is self-sustaining. The individuals will most often be reclusive, eating to relieve themselves of grief when grief itself is what prompts them to indulge.

2. Stress Eating

People react to pressure in many different ways. At the same time, some deny themselves of life's pleasures when they are under duress. Others will indulge themselves with utter abandon to either cope with or distract their thoughts from stressful situations. It is the latter that are susceptible to stress eating.

Anxiety and stress eating are directly related to the production of cortisol, also known as the stress hormone. When an individual is under duress, cortisol is sent into the body, where it blurs reason, forcing people to overreact to their circumstance. For those that indulge in food as a reaction to stress, the jump in their serotonin (happy hormone) levels provides momentary relief. The aftermath, however, is quite the opposite. Once the sugar fades from their bloodstream, the individual moves from their temporary 'high' to a relative low, feeling tired or depressed.

3. Binge Eating

This is one of the most dangerous characteristics of sugar addiction because its effects are especially telling. The overall effects on mental and emotional health are sinister and complex. The individual will often eat too much, too fast, and at a stretch with far-reaching implications. Aside from the concern of obesity, there's the associated issue of dwindled self-worth coupled with a crippling sense of shame and disgust for oneself.

4. Withdrawal Symptoms

When someone who is addicted stops taking sugar, just like with any substance, they will begin to have withdrawal symptoms. They might experience moodiness, loss of strength, and irritability. The longevity of the symptoms varies from person to person; however, the effects are often quite intense when you consider that people who struggle with sugar addiction binge on it.

5. Alcoholism

In a shocking discovery, a 2003 study at Mt. Sinai School of Medicine revealed a direct genetic link between parents who abused alcohol and children with sugar addiction. The findings showed how the dopamine receptors in the alcoholic parent's brain lit up similarly to the ones in the brains of their children as they enjoyed a sugary snack. The implication is alcoholic parents can pass down genes to their children, leaving them with a much higher tendency to get addicted to sugar.

Already established is the fact that individuals who regularly consume alcohol are more inclined to consume sugary substances. Although this is genetic and something people have total control over, it helps to note if you or any other person might be a victim of your previous generation's choices.

Why Sugar Addiction Is A Problem In America

The 20th century saw the rise of consumerism and the evolution of sugar. What is now endemic to Americans' lives was once viewed as a triumph and herald of more to come. Needless to say, the 'more' has finally come, and it is a rising revolution against the devastating consequences of sugar consumption. It's no secret that the statistics look especially bleak.

In America today, only 30% of its citizens are classified as having a healthy weight, and around a third of children are generally considered either obese or overweight. Despite the massive budget set aside every year for dealing with weight-related diseases, the rate of diabetes in the country has not slowed. In fact, it has actually increased. Medical researchers are finally beginning to agree that sugar is the problem.

America has a long and deep tradition with sugar. It is reflected in almost every part of its society, its culture, and how citizens have come to relate with it. There are billion-dollar corporations that are dedicated to creating and serving different types of confectioneries that are all sugar-based. These, of course, include commonly marketed donuts, burgers and soft drinks. Movie theaters and sporting events have their own unwritten rule of what entails a satisfactory experience, which always includes sugary popcorn, salty snacks, and high fructose soda. Amusement parks and outdoor festivities also peddle sugar in every snack, drink, or food you buy on their grounds. National holidays, such as Halloween, also contribute to the epidemic through the tradition of sharing candy.

Almost every American is a devoted client to a soda brand whose sugar content is far from safe. Statistics also report that the average child will drink at least one cup of soda every day and it increases as they age into adulthood. To top this statistic, studies concluded that, in a year, the average American adult consumess at least 170 liters of sugar-based drinks, which doubles that of Europeans.

One defining factor that makes it very easy for anyone to abuse sugar is its discreet nature. An average bottle of name brand soda contains up to 16 tsp of sugar, which is more than twice the recommended amount advised for women and double the amount suggested for men. To make matters worse, you will hardly notice how many bottles you consume because soft drinks neither satiate hunger nor quench thirst.

As I mentioned earlier, this revealing information means nothing when you consider how addictive sugar actually is. Coupled with its legality and widespread acceptance, it is one of the most formidable foes our overall health will ever face, mostly because many people are in denial of its adverse effects.

Recently, leading medical experts agreed that sugar might be as addictive as cocaine.[1]. While this might sound like an outlandish statement, it is not in any way far from the truth when you closely examine the way sugar works on a behavioral and hormonal level.

So how do you get a country to break their addiction?

The truth is, the country as a whole, must work together to battle the crisis. Consumers, food manufacturers, and the government, must all recognize the problem sugar poses on a national scale. Considering the complex web of our dependencies, corporate interest, and the economic fallout of such a task, it should come as no surprise that this is where the problem begins and the solution likely ends.

How High Sugar Diets Damage Your Health

Sugar tastes great but when you consume too much, it becomes harmful to your health. Aside from obesity, excess sugar consumption has been known to lead to heart disease, which can contribute to premature death. Excess consumption also weakens the body's immune system, causes sleepless nights and produces inflammation. Since the body's immune system is the major defense system that protects you from falling ill too frequently, increased inflammation makes it more difficult to heal from any injury or infection that may occur. It can also make you hypertensive, and overweight. When you are in this condition, you tend to be unhealthy and unwilling to exercise because of your drop in energy levels.

Beyond the major issues just mentioned, a myriad of other negative side effects can occur. The following list should allow you to understand more explicitly, how detrimental overconsumption can be to your health.

1. High sugar consumption causes the body's glucose levels to rise and fall erratically, resulting in extreme fatigue, frequent mood swings, and splitting headaches.

2. Overconsumption greatly increases the risk of diabetes, heart disease, and obesity.

3. Sugar has also been identified as one of the accelerators of aging. When consuming sugar, it directly attaches to proteins in the body's bloodstream. A chemical reaction then occurs which adversely affects the skin's elasticity and causes it to sag, which leads to premature aging.

4. A well-known but often disregarded side effect is sugar's effect on the teeth. It causes plaque, cavities, and tooth decay. While this might not be life-threatening, it still detracts from your overall well-being.

5. Sugar can cause chronic gum infections, which can also lead to heart disease. The connection was drawn from our body system's inflammatory reaction to infection.

6. High sugar consumption also affects brain function. Of all the points on this bleak list, the most heartbreaking is how sugar can affect children's cognition. A study in New York City public schools tested sugar's relation to cognition by removing sugar from their classroom rewards. The result was that researchers saw a startling 15.7% increase in academic performance.

CASE STUDY: THE LITTLE ISLAND OF TOKELAU

To illustrate how destructive a sugar-centric diet is, let's take a look at a small island nation called Tokelau.

In the 1960's, Tokelau's regional diet had only 2% of its calories coming from sugar and 50% from fat, which was mostly saturated. It consisted mainly of fish, coconut, chicken, breadfruit, and pork, where only a relatively minuscule 9% of Tokelauan women and about 3% of Tokelauan men had diabetes.

However, 50 years later and after a dramatic rise in the adoption of the West's sugar-saturated diet, Tokelau now has the highest rate of diabetes by population density of any country in the world. In 2014, 38% of all the nation's population had diabetes and now more than two-thirds of Tokelau island is obese. This, if nothing else in this chapter, is practical proof of the adverse effects of sugar on the human body and our health.

KEY POINTS

In this chapter, you have learned about the warning signs and effects of a sugar addiction. Here are a few takeaways:

- One of the quickest signs of sugar addiction in a person is overeating.
- Alcoholism is often overlooked and can also be a cause of sugar addiction.
- Binge eating, Stress eating, and Withdrawal symptoms are all precise characteristics and signs of sugar addiction.
- America's sugar problem can be linked to its sugar-reliant culture.
- Aside from tooth decay, fluctuating glucose levels, and obesity, sugar has also been proven to adversely affect children's cognition.
- The little Island of Tokelau saw a serious increase in cases of diabetes after adopting western sugar-based diets.

We have dealt extensively with the adverse effects of sugar on our body system. You have learned the realities of its addictive properties and the national, global celebrity status it enjoys despite its destructive qualities. However, just like all things, the problem lies in overuse. Sugar is not a total villain. In fact, our body still needs sugar to function, and a lot of the carbohydrates we eat do just that. In the next chapter, I am going to show you how to identify what sugar is both good and harmful to you.

2. The Truth About Good And Bad Sugars

Various foods that fall under similar classes sometimes contain different types of sugars. That's why it's no surprise that some foods of the same classes are acceptable on a diet, while others are not. The various sugars obtained from the body are eventually broken down into glucose. However, how do we identify which is beneficial to our health and which will cause potential harm to the body? How can we discover what type of sugar is needed for our body's metabolism? Both of these questions will be answered in this chapter to help you balance your sugar intake.

How Is Sugar Healthy?

Nearly every food (natural or processed) comprises some form of natural or added sugars. For the purposes of a detox, the sugars you should reduce and, most preferably, avoid are added sugars. They are directly linked to obesity, type II diabetes, high blood pressure, inflammation and heart disease.

However, not all sugars are prone to make you vulnerable to these health conditions. Do you think the sugars found in a blended cup of berries are similar to that from a bottle of cola? If your answer is yes, then keep reading, as I will quickly help you see the differences between natural and added sugars.

Natural Sugars & Their Sources

Simply put, natural sugars are the ones found in natural, unprocessed food items. Irrespective of what we're lead to believe by food processing marketers, natural sugars can only be found in two forms- lactose and frustose. Lactose is found in milk and diary, while fructose is found in most, if not all, common fruits.

Food items rich in natural sugars are known to have the purest form of carbohydrates safe for ingestion. By the same token, the direct food source of these carbohydrates is known to offer even more nutritional benefits. Milk and edible fruits, for instance, supply the body considerable amounts of vitamin A, protein, fiber, calcium, vitamin C, and vitamin D.

More importantly, foods with natural sugars are known to be significantly high sources of minerals while being low in sodium and calories. Fiber, which is often obtained from fruits, allows the body to digest food quick and easy. This, in turn, prevents the expected sugar rush from consuming a doughnut, which would otherwise lead to constipation. Lactose derived from milk also provides the body with a sustainable amount of energy, keeping you filled longer than the sugars from a typical bottle of soda. Fibers are a great source for sustained energy and provide the body with a better satiety value.

We just looked at natural sugars (which are also known as simple sugars) and their sources. These are the kinds of sugars recommended for daily intake because of their overall nourishing importance to the body. Naturally occurring sugars benefit your health more because of their components rich in minerals, phytochemicals, vitamins, fiber, and protein. The benefits attached to fiber make natural sugars healthier and more beneficial than processed sugars. Fiber in natural sugars also helps reduce the absorption of carbohydrates in the body. When the absorption action of sugar is slowed down, the significance of blood sugar is reduced.

What Are Added Sugars, Exactly?

Added sugars, in basic terms, are sweeteners added to processed foods and drinks. They are "added" to make food better tasting. These sugars are mostly found in carbonated drinks, cakes, candies, cookies and several sugary processed foods. Most people end up consuming more added sugar than the national recommended daily limit.

Added sugars are far from healthy because they contain a high amount of calories, which could lead to increased blood pressure and the risk of heart disease. These sugars are known to replace nutritious-dense foods in your blood making your body deprived of its required nutrients.

To make matters worse, added sugars increase the caloric intake to your diet, causing weight gain. Granulated sugar, maple syrup, and other types of sweeteners are processed and manufactured to be food additives to sweeten the taste. Sometimes, the degree of sweetness varies among all types, but in the end they contain at least 14 calories per teaspoon. Over time, this intake accumulates and leads to weight gain since added sugars only provide excess calories. Therefore, it is best to focus on consuming only healthy calories to provide your body with essential nutrients.

Added Sugars Daily Recommended Limit

While it is no mystery that added sugars cause more harm than good, people with underlying medical issues also consume them. Patients with low blood sugar are advised by medical doctors to adopt the intake of added sugars for supplements. When taken as prescribed, these patients could level up their blood sugar level and keep it normal over time. That being said, people without medical conditions need to be aware of the recommended daily limit on added sugars.

Medical professionals now recommend that no more than fifty percent of your total daily calorie intake should come from added sugars. This recommended limit varies in men and women, as the bodies of both genders react differently to sugar consumption. The limits were previously mentioned at the beginning of this book, but they are definitely worth repeating:

- For men, the recommended limit is 9 teaspoons of added sugars, which is an equivalent of 150 calories daily.
- For women, the recommended limit is 6 teaspoons, which equates to 100 calories daily.

A Quick Note: Many people believe that high-fructose corn syrup isn't a part of the added sugar group and this recommendation doesn't apply. This couldn't be any further from the truth as high-fructose corn syrup is most definitely an added sugar and should be carefully ingested.

The Short Term Effects of Added Sugars

Food manufacturers include added sugars to their product formulas to help sweeten the taste of their brand. However, processed foods rich in added sugars like drinks, cookies, and cakes cause more health problems to the body when consumed outside of the daily recommended limit. To review, let's recap the four top medical reasons why added sugars are unhealthy:

- **Low Nutritional Value:** Added sugars are sources of empty calories, which do not provide the body with any nutrients. They are also not reliable for sustained energy as the body breaks them down quickly. On the other hand, foods containing natural sugars are digested by the body at a slower rate and offer sustained energy.

- **Weight Gain:** The increased consumption of added sugars could lead to weight gain over a short period. Even with exercise, eating foods that contain high levels of added sugars will still inhibit your weight loss goals.

- **Diabetes:** The exessive intake of added sugars has a direct link to type II diabetes. It's important to note, however, that sugar intake isn't the only cause of diabetes. Diets high in saturated fat also lead to type II diabetes. However, sugary drinks have been connected first-hand to those diagnosed with the disease.

- **Tooth Cavities:** The quickest source of tooth decay and further cavity issues can be traced to the high intake of sugar. When we ingest sugar, the bacteria found in the mouth react with the sugar particles to form an acid harmful to the teeth. Even though the body has a defense mechanism in place to repair damaged parts of the teeth, excess sugar consumption leads to lasting deterioration.

The Long Term Effects of Added Sugars

If the short-term effects aren't bad enough, the long-term effects of high sugar consumption are even worse. As previously mentioned, added sugars are known to be the root cause of several severe ailments and diseases. While reading this frightening list, you will see just how important a sugar detox is for your body.

- **Skin Aging**: The human skin has components made up of collagen and elastin, which are responsible for the tenderness, supple nature and softness of the skin. Excess added sugars have been known to cause the collagen to get cross-linked. When this occurs on multiple spots of the skin, elastin loses its effectiveness, which leads to stiffness on the skin's surface. This process eventually results in skin aging.

- **Cardiovascular Disease**: Type II diabetes, which has been linked to excess added sugars, often results in cardiovascular diseases. A sudden spike or increase in blood sugar levels over time leads to heart disease and obesity.

- **Colon Cancer**: Excessive consumption of added sugars could cause inflammation, which in turn leads to various cancerous growths in the body. The colon is one of the first areas of the human body to react to inflammation, which results in colon cancer.

- **High Blood Pressure**: Added sugars increase the formation of uric acid, which causes a spike in the overall blood pressure of the body. Excessive intake of added sugars also reduces the production of Nitric Oxide in blood vessels, which is a vital component in maintaining the elasticity level of each blood vessel. When its production is affected, the blood vessels become congested which directly affects blood pressure.

- **Kidney Disease**: Similar to increased blood pressure, excessive consumption of added sugars could cause damage in the blood vessels of the kidney. Most kidney diseases stem from the irregular flow of blood into the organ. When high blood pressure in the kidney isn't diagnosed early enough, kidney failure can occur.

- **Liver Disease**: The liver utilizes fructose in its regular production of fat. When you stock up on excess added sugar and mostly high-fructose corn syrup, an enormous production of fat in the liver occurs. This common fat build-up is what leads to liver diseases.

- **Obesity**: A regular excessive intake of added sugars results in a build-up of leptin resistance, increased blood sugar, and insulin resistance. All these occurances combined lead to the production of excess body fat.

- **Pancreatic Cancer**: Added sugars in the blood affects the regulated production of insulin, which is responsible for growing and dividing of the pancreas cells. With excessive sugar intake, the production of insulin becomes irregular in the blood. This imbalance of insulin can result in cancerous cells growing and spreading throughout the pancreas.

How Added Sugars Create Addiction

As you are probably aware, regular consumption of added sugars can be addictive. The human tongue is quite responsive to sweet taste, more so than bitterness. Added sugar addiction isn't hereditary, but it can be developed at a young age. Adults who find it difficult to refrain from foods rich in added sugars often do not have a taste for anything else. They are so used to the daily intake of soft drinks, cakes and cookies, that they need to satisfy these cravings regularly.

When added sugar addiction is established, it takes committed effort to reverse it. Fortunately, the human body learns to adjust to a healthier diet over time, which is why it is advisable that you feed your body with the right foods. Once a healthy diet is part of your daily routine, you won't feel stresssed about avoiding added sugars.

How To Quickly Identify Added Sugar on Labels

We're easily deceived nowadays with products tagged as "zero sugar". Before you pick them up during your next visit to the grocery store, it is important to read this section carefully. Processed foods like instant oatmeal, baby food, pasta sauces, protein bars, cereal, ketchup and salad dressings all fall under the categories of foods with added sugar. It's almost impossible to produce these food items without including them in their formulas. Foods like granola, barbecue sauces and flavored yogurt also fall in the same category.

In the market nowadays, checking the labels isn't as simple as it used to be. We now have sugars being swapped with several names that might be extremely difficult to spot by a consumer. For nutritional labels, you should be on the look out for corn syrup, maltose, malt syrup, rice syrup, high-fructose corn syrup, maple syrup, and virtually any "syrup-inclusive" ingredient.

Added sugar can also be disguised by a few more terms, so check labels for the following:

- Barley malt
- Brown sugar
- Invert sugar
- Trehalose
- Corn sweetner
- Raw sugar
- Lactose
- Sucrose
- Honey

Likewise, the following ingredients are less common high sugar identifiers:

- Fructose
- Dextrose
- Molasses
- Glucose
- Pancake syrup
- Turbinado sugar

With this list of nutritional labels, you should be able to spot food items with added sugars more quickly and easily. We can avoid the health damage caused by added sugars by sticking to the recommended sugar daily limit. If you've never been cautious about this before, it might take a lot of commitment on your part. Nonetheless, it ultimately pays off because it helps you stay healthy.

In this chapter, we've looked at the healthy and unhealthy aspects of sugar. You learned about the kinds of sugars beneficial to your body, as well as, the dangers of added sugars. You also learned about the extensive damage added sugars could cause on your health. Lastly, I shared tips on how to identify foods high in added sugar. It is my sincere hope that this chapter helps you make better health decisions after reading.

But what if you've already fallen victim to an excessive sugar intake? What if your doctor just confirmed that you are overweight? Is this book only intended for prevention? Certainly, not. The next chapter serves as a complete guide on how to start a successful sugar detox, where you will learn all the steps to relieveing your body from excess added sugar.

Ready? Turn the next page and let's get started!

3. How To Start A Successful Sugar Detox

It is important to note that that topic of this chapter includes the word "successful", since there are both successful and unsuccessful ways to complete a sugar detox. This book aims to avoid a case where you start your sugar detox program and throw in the towel after a few hours. This typically occurs when a person's withdrawal symptoms kick in within the first 24 hours. Using myself as an example, my first sugar detox program lasted for less than a day. As I remember it now, I can look back and laugh at myself, even though the struggle was very emotional at the time. In this chapter, I will talk more about some of my failed sugar detox experiences before I finally got it right.

To help you start and successfully complete your sugar detox program without a hitch and I will be shedding more light on the following concepts:

- What a sugar detox is.

- Your body's reaction to successful sugar detox therapy.

- The benefits of a sugar detox to your overall health.

- How to change your diet.

- The best foods items for your sugar detox plan.

- Ideas for both a 5-day and 7-day sugar detox meal plan.

As you can see, this chapter is a big one, where you have a lot to learn. So sit back, relax, and join me as I guide you on your path to breaking your sugar addiction!

What is A Sugar Detox?

A sugar detox is a process whereby an individual flushes their body of excess and unwanted sugar. This process, however, is not an easy feat for most. Since your body is used to being fed with a high sugar intake, cutting off and reducing these intakes may have you experiencing side effects, which can last for a few days.

Withdrawal symptoms can include any of the following:

- Fatigue
- Difficulty in concentration
- Dizziness
- Anxiety
- Headaches
- Mood swings and irritation
- Insomnia
- Depression

Keeping these symptoms in mind, the benefits of a successful sugar detox are quite shocking. Aside from the obvious victory of you breaking your sugar addiction, here are the most important:

- **Fat Loss**

As previously discussed, added sugars create unwanted fat in the body, most especially in the belly and waist area. When you reduce your intake of added sugar, fat gained during your sugar binge will reduce drastically.

• **A Reduction in Food Cravings**

As a sugar addict, your cravings for food and drinks will be high as you will always have the urge to eat something every hour of the day. These cravings will reduce to a minimum when you are on a sugar detox. As a result of your conscious sugar abstinence and your new intake of healthy foods, you will stay filled, and have little to no sugar cravings.

• **Hormonal Balancing**

Excess intake of sugar is a prime suspect of hormonal imbalance, most especially in women. This is why you find that women who eat too much added sugar experience terrible PMS and irregular periods. A decrease in sugar intake will help balance these hormones, such that PMS is reduced and monthly periods become regular.

• **Decreased Brain Inflammation**

Excess sugar consumption causes brain inflammation, such that the spinal cord and brain cells become inflamed and irritated. This can be reversed by a decline in added sugar intake.

• **Reduces Risk of Chronic Diseases**

Excess added sugar is one of the key factors that affect an individual's body system and causes the body to degenerate. This degeneration can lead to some chronic diseases such as cardiovascular, kidney, and liver diseases, gouts, cancer, and diabetes. Cutting back on sugar to give room for healthy and nutritious food will help mitigate the risks of these diseases and help keep the body, mind, and soul healthy.

• **Healthy Teeth**

The more you binge on sugar, the more your teeth get robbed of the useful minerals that are meant to keep them strong and healthy. With a sugar addiction lifestyle, the hard tissues of the teeth such as the cementum, dentine, and enamel will begin to experience dissolution, erosion, and cavitation. When you stop ingesting sugary food items, you will find that your teeth will become healthy again as they regain their lost materials through a process known as "tooth remineralization".

Food Characteristics Of A Sugar Detox

Sugar detoxification isn't just about staying away from sugar. It is focused on altering your sugar-addicted diet and replacing it with a healthy and nutritious one. The following list includes some of the best food items that you need on a successful sugar detox journey.

- **Healthy Oil/Fats**

These include wholesome oils (such as olive and coconut oil), seeds, nuts, cheese, and dark chocolate.

- **Low-glycemic index (GI) foods**

Low GI value food items are important in living a healthy lifestyle since they are slowly digested into the body, thereby ensuring that the blood sugar is reduced. Foods with low GI value include oats, milk, wholegrain bread, quinoa, yogurt, and pasta.

- **Protein**

Including protein food items such as chicken, legumes, fish, lamb, beef, egg, soy, quinoa, and oatmeal, help to promote a feeling of fullness so that you won't feel hungry over an extended period of time.

- **Fruits**

Fruits contain antioxidants, minerals, and vitamins that help you digest food properly, improve your outward appearance, and also boost sugar detoxification successfully. The types of fruits that you can include in your diet as desserts or smoothies include oranges, grapefruit, lemons, pawpaws, apples, and berries.

- **Healthy Carbs**

To ensure a successful sugar detox plan, you need to boycott starchy and unhealthy carbs and focus on healthy carbs such as brown rice, white potatoes, whole grains, and whole cereals amongst others.

- **Vegetables**

Broccoli, cabbage, fennel, cauliflower, kale, and spinach are some of the best vegetables to include in your sugar detox program. These vegetables will help fight against toxins in the body, mitigate blood pressure and cholesterol levels, while also boosting your immune system.

- **Water**

To replace your carbonated drinks, stick with sparkling water, plain water, fruit-infused water, healthy smoothies, and unsweetened herbal tea to ensure that you stay hydrated.

Aside from indulging in the previously mentioned food items, there are other activities that you need to engage in to ensure that your sugar detox plan will proceed successfully.

- Rest well

Getting good rest when necessary is another way through which you can revive lost energy. It also helps to reduce sugar while helping to mitigate hormones that trigger food cravings.

- Engage in exercise

Engaging in exercises will help to release endorphin hormones, which are hormones that will give you that same feel-good emotion that sugar provides. Exercising also helps to lower sugar levels, and mitigate the effects of sugar withdrawal symptoms to a minimum.

• Reduce your stress levels

Undergoing too much stress can have you craving sugary food items to boost your energy and keep you active. In a case when you reduce the amount of stress that you undergo on a daily basis, you will see that your craving for sugary food items will reduce and you will feel less stressed as a result.

My Experience With A Sugar Detox Program

Prior to attempting my first detox, my sugar addiction was focused on chocolates, cookies, and carbonated drinks. My love for these items was second to none. It was not unusual for me to eat at least 5 bars of chocolates, cookies, while gulping down at least 2 bottles of carbonated drink in one day. Needless to say, my addiction was off the charts.

At that point, I had convinced myself that I was just merely suffering from a sweet tooth. I mean, who doesn't suffer from one every once in a while? So I continued this unhealthy consumption of cookies, carbonated drinks, and chocolate, and the while, feeling like it was a normal thing to do.

Fast forward to a couple of months later, and I noticed that my ingestion of these things had doubled in quantity. I was on a regular "diet" of at least 4 carbonated drinks, 10 chocolate bars, and 5 cookie packs a day! This should have made me scared, right? Nope. The truth was, I still didn't see anything wrong with my habits. I figured that as a writer who spent most of her time working her brain cells out, I needed the sugar to maintain my energy each day.

For me, binging was a good excuse. I continued like that for another couple of months until my moment of epiphany arrived when I found out that I was doing more harm to myself than good. Each time I binged on these things, I felt an immediate surge of energy, but within a few minutes, my energy and body completely crashed. This, in turn, would cause me to binge harder and harder, until I crossed the threshold of indulging in cravings, to actually being addicted to the foods in order to get my work done. Even worse, this experience coupled with insomnia, a bout of depression and feeling emotionally imbalanced, led me to rethink my diet. Luckily, I had the trust and confidence of a close friend to help me start to change.

My friend had been a dietician for many years and immediately made me get rid of all my chocolate bars, cookie packs, and carbonated drinks. On the first day, I packed all these dangerous culprits and tossed them in a kitchen cupboard which I locked and hid the key. I had water after my breakfast, and at different intervals in the morning, but by noon, I couldn't take it anymore. I found my "hidden" key and opened the kitchen cabinet and grabbed all my sugary snacks and had a go at them again. Looking back on myself in that moment, I felt like a failure.

This occurred more times than I can count. After so many unsuccessful attempts, I forgot a key component of a successful sugar detox that my friend advised me on. I learned that getting in a sugar detox plan doesn't mean I cut out my sugar cravings all at once, but I should *replace* my sugar cravings with healthier items.

It was at that point, that I started snacking on healthy energy bars in place of the regular chocolate. I had fruit and vegetable smoothies in place of the carbonated drinks. I made my own low sugar oatmeal based cookies instead of consuming the unhealthy store bought ones. Before long, I broke up with my sugar addiction, and the effects on my body were incredible.

If you are a sugar junkie like I was, it is essential that I warn you that a sugar detox is not going to be easy, as you could face many physical, psychological, and emotional challenges during your withdrawal phase. Not everyone reacts the same, but you could experience mental and physiological symptoms such as mood swings, depression, digestive issues, restlessness, and a lack of energy. This means that you have to brace yourself for what could occur in the short term.

Preparing for a Sugar Detox

Now that you've taken your first step towards completing a proper sugar detox, you must understand the importance of preparation. As Benjamin Franklin's saying goes: "If you fail to plan, you are planning to fail!" Getting yourself into the right mindset is essential, but you also need to do a few tangible and physical things to start yourself off on the right foot.

Clean Out Your Fridge and Pantry

This first step may be difficult. You need to go through your fridge and pantry and remove everything—and I mean *everything*—that contains sugar. It can be super easy to justify not doing it because if we're just throwing away food, it's a waste, right? Wrong. It's up to you to find something useful to do with that food. Give it away or take it to an organization that needs it.

Plan Your Meals Ahead of Time

One of the biggest dangers people face is getting to dinnertime and not knowing what to cook or eat. The other big problem is visiting someone else and not knowing if there's sugar in what they're feeding you. When it comes to cooking, I plan for a week and make sure I have all the ingredients I need upfront. You can even cook in advance if you're good with meal prep.

Another big part of planning your meals in advance is covering what to do if you're at a restaurant or visiting a friend. Most menus have a reasonably straightforward option that should be mostly sugar-free, and most friends or family should understand and cater accordingly.

Stay Hydrated

Did you know that dehydration is often mistaken for hunger? Keeping on top of your hydration is extremely important to keep you feeling full and not craving sugar. The average adult man needs 15 glasses of water a day. Women need about 12.

Are you getting that much water in? Challenge yourself to work your way up to it; you may be surprised at how many fewer cravings you get. If you struggle with plain old water, then try carbonated water. The bubbles do wonders for helping you feel full.

Get Enough Sleep

This has been said before, but it is worth repeating. Sleep is another enemy of a sugar detox. When you're tired, your brain does this funny thing where it tricks your body into craving sugar. Sugar quickly absorbs into the body, which gives us a speedy burst of energy when the body is tired. However, it also wears off quickly, leaving us feeling worse (and more hungry) than before. Getting enough sleep means your body isn't constantly searching for something to ingest to give it energy.

Foods to Avoid

Unfortunately, giving up sugar means you *will* need to sacrifice some foods. There's just no getting around it. If you're serious about kicking the sugar habit, then making healthy choices is what you need to do. Sure, it's going to be tough—you'll be tempted to cheat. However, you won't succeed if you don't commit to it; part of committing to your goal is avoiding things that contain the sweet temptations.

If you're unwilling to take this step, you may need to put this book down and spend some time considering your health. If you're on board and ready to make a lasting change, here's what you should be avoiding:

Processed Foods

Processed foods are often treated with chemical ingredients to make them stay fresher for longer. Standard-processed foods like bread and cheese include ingredients you wouldn't normally find in your average kitchen; however, the more dangerous ultra-processed foods contain a variety of additives that can be detrimental to a sugar detox.

These ingredients often come with their own side effects, but the biggest issue comes in when food manufacturers add extra sugar to their products to mask the flavors of these additives. To give you an indication of how big a problem this is, a study concluded that heavily processed foods make up 60% of total food, and 90% of the sugars we consume come from these foods.

Added Sugar

It goes without saying that eating foods with added sugar will ruin a sugar detox. Many processed foods contain sugar to cover up the bitter taste caused by other additives. It's also super easy to hide. You may not see "sugar" on an ingredient list; what you might find are ingredients like dextrose, fructose, glucose and sucrose. Other names for sugar (in various forms) include corn syrup, dextrin, ethyl maltol, Florida crystals, maltodextrin, sucanat, agave, molasses, carob, or treacle.

Refined Carbohydrates & Sugars

Refined carbs and sugars are often found in processed foods. These are 'simple carbs' and include refined white flour, white rice, pasta, and cereals. Refined sugars can be found in things like flavored yogurt, fruit juices, salad dressing, and pasta sauces.

They're absorbed quickly but have little nutritional value, so you'll be hungry again in an hour. This can lead to cravings that are hard to deal with when you're doing a sugar detox.

Sodium Nitrite & Nitrate

These additives are most commonly added to processed meat and are used to give it color and increase its shelf life. They're also found naturally in many vegetables, and their addition to processed meat can have negative health effects, including an increased risk of colorectal cancer (Cantwell & Elliott, 2017).

The biggest danger that these contribute to a sugar detox is that sugar is often added to counteract their flavor and make the meat more palatable. Specific foods to avoid are as follows:

- Hot dog sausages
- Salami
- Corned beef
- Ham
- Beef jerky
- Frozen dinners
- Granola bars
- Canned foods
- Instant noodles
- Most breakfast cereals

High-Sugar Vegetables

Yes, even some vegetables are extremely sugary. This isn't refined sugar—it's natural. However, it can still push your body's sugar levels up too much; if you're serious about detoxing, it's a good idea to leave them off your plate.

When completing a detox, it is best to avoid the following:

- White potatoes
- Sweet potatoes
- Beetroot
- Peas
- Corn
- Chickpeas
- Onion
- Parsnips
- Red bell peppers

All of these vegetables have more than 4 grams of sugar per 100 grams of the food. The good news is there are still plenty more vegetables you can eat, so get creative when it comes to cooking them.

Takeout

When you order a takeout meal, you have no idea what it's been prepared with. For example, even something as plain as fish and chips could have sugar in the fish fries' batter. Ordering an entree like a steak or chicken breast may seem safe, but even they've been marinated in some kind of sauce, so there's really no way of telling.

If you end up going to a function and you can't steer clear of restaurant food, that's okay for one meal. But, if you're staying home and ordering in because you don't feel like cooking, that's not going to go well with a sugar detox.

Sauces & Dressings

You may think you can get by with no sugar simply by adding a dash of dressing to your salad or making a tasty and healthy pasta dish. Eating simple, tasty meals will prevent those sweet cravings, right? The truth is, a salad coated in dressing or a saucy pasta could help reduce cravings, but only because your salad dressing and pasta sauce most likely has sugar in it.

Salad Dressing

Salad dressings contain sugar in varying quantities, so if you're going completely sugar-free you'd need to avoid them all. Fat-free salad dressings are the worst culprits because they contain more than three times that of normal dressings. Removing fat causes an unsavory taste, so extra sugar is added to counteract that. You can be as good as you want with your food, but it really doesn't help your detox if you're eating salad every day and coating it in sugary dressing.

Sauces

Pasta sauces, marinades, and meat sauces may be savory, but manufacturers add sugar to curb the acidity of ingredients such as tomato. Take note of the ingredient list: some sauces list corn syrup instead of sugar. It's wise to buy a sugar-free version or make your own if you're serious about a sugar detox. Be wary of ketchup, pasta sauce, pizza sauce, meat sauce, mayonnaise, sweet chili sauce, pesto, mustard, and brown sauces.

Dried or Canned Fruit

When we eat dried fruit, we don't just have one piece. Fruit is generally healthy and a source of natural sugars, but when it's dried, it concentrates all that sugar into a tiny bite. On top of the natural sugars raw fruit contains, dried fruit can be tart when the hydration is removed, so they're often sprinkled with powdered sugar or have added liquid sugar. It can be easy to forget that dried fruits contain sugar, as they're touted as a healthy snack option. It can also be very easy to overdo it and end up eating many more calories and sugars than you intended to.

As for canned fruit, it's often canned in heavy syrup. Even if it's canned in its own juice, it can be difficult to be sure that there's no added sugar. It's best to stick to fresh, whole fruits.

Soft Drinks & Fruit Juice (Packaged)

We all know that soda is laced with sugar, and even "sugar-free" drinks are loaded with unhealthy sweeteners that can actually make you crave more. But did you know that fruit juice is just as loaded? That 'healthy' drink is really just another sugar high hidden in fruity packaging. If you've ever tried drinking freshly squeezed fruit juice, you'll know that it's not usually as sweet as store-bought drinks. In fact, it can sometimes be quite sour. Can you see why manufacturers add sugar?

In addition to added sugars, there's a lot of natural sugar in a glass of fruit juice. In fact, one serving of fruit juice can contain the calories and sugars of up to three fruits, so drinking it elevates your sugar levels far more than you realize.

Low-Fat Foods

Research has found that the sugar content of low-fat foods is higher than in normal foods. The most sugar-saturated, low-fat foods include dairy products, baked goods, meat, fats and oils, margarine, butter, and salad dressings (Nguyen et al., 2016). There's a simple reason for this: when you remove fat from a food, the end result is an unappealing taste. Manufacturers add sugar to make the food more palatable.

It's hard to find tasty foods that are both fat-free and sugar-free. It's best to avoid fat-free foods, as you may be accidentally eating something that's extra high in sugar. This goes for diary foods like low-fat yogurt, low-fat cheese and low-fat milk.

Alcohol

Most alcohol is almost pure sugar. Mixed drinks, especially, have added flavors, which pushes them way over the limit of how much sugar we should be ingesting. Limiting your alcohol intake—or giving it up for the course of your detox—is a good way to drastically lower your sugar intake.

Foods to Eat

Now that you're aware of what you shouldn't be eating, what's left? The good news is that there are plenty of high-quality, healthy items for us to be making meals out of. In this section, we'll be focusing on whole foods that have been minimally processed and contain a low amount of sugar.

Lean Proteins

Proteins are nutrient-dense, so they take longer to digest than carbs do. This means they keep you feeling fuller for longer. You won't be getting cravings because you're eating empty calories, so you're more likely to stick to your sugar detox.

Eat a bit of protein with every meal to reap the benefits. They're also packed with healthy amino acids and are all low in sugar, but you won't miss the sweet stuff if you're eating healthy, nutrient-dense meals.

As well as getting your fill of amino acids that the body needs, research suggests that protein doesn't raise blood glucose levels by much. Those with type 2 diabetes who are looking to go on a sugar detox would benefit enormously from eating lean proteins, as evidence shows that blood glucose levels actually drop after eating a high-protein meal.

Examples of lean proteins include:

- Chicken & turkey (frozen or uncooked)
- Beef (ground beef is fine, marinated is not)
- Fish (try to avoid battered fish: go for white-fleshed)
- Pork
- Bison
- Egg whites

Low-Sugar Vegetables

Eating vegetables is important to keep your vitamin, mineral, and antioxidant levels up. Deficiencies caused by low-nutrition foods (empty calories) can enhance sugar cravings. Getting a daily dose of vegetables keeps your levels where they should be and reduces the chance of your body accidentally interpreting a vitamin deficiency as a sugar craving. Keep in mind that you don't only need to cook and eat vegetables with dinner. Things like celery, cucumber, soybean sprouts, lettuce, radishes, and Swiss chard all make the list of top 15 lowest sugar vegetables, and you could make a super salad with them.

Broccoli, spinach, brussel sprouts, carrots, eggplant, zucchini, cabbage, and yellow peppers are just a few of the options you can add to your plate every single day. Try not to stick to only green veggies. You want a combination of colors to make sure you get all the necessary antioxidants and nutrients from them. If you're a fan of smoothies, you can even add some low-sugar veggies to your smoothie at breakfast. It's not hard to get your daily dose if you think creatively.

Fruits

Mangoes, dates, and pineapple should be avoided as they're high in sugar; everything else is free game. Don't worry about the natural sugars in the fruit, as they're not high enough to be a problem. In fact, noshing on a piece of fruit could be exactly what you need when the sugar cravings hit. It should be enough to satisfy your sweet need, without the negative side effects that processed sugar leaves behind. As well as tackling your sweet craving, you'll be getting a dose of vitamins, minerals, and antioxidants that you wouldn't get in a candy bar.

The next time a sugar craving hits you, reach for one of these fruits of these instead of a processed sugary snack:

- Raspberries (5g natural sugar per cup)
- Strawberries (7-8g natural sugar per cup)
- Blackberries (7g natural sugar per cup)
- Cranberries (4.7g natural sugar per cup)
- Watermelon (10g natural sugar per cup)
- Kiwi (6g natural sugar per fruit)
- Starfruit (4.3g natural sugar per cup)
- Plum (7g natural sugar per fruit)

Whole Wheat Pasta & Grains

Whole wheat foods may seem boring in comparison to their processed cousins, but they're by far the healthier option, and may be lower in sugar too! Whole wheat pasta and bread are acceptable to eat on a sugar detox. You may see 'low GI' on their packaging. This means that the body takes longer to absorb them, so there's no rapid spike in blood sugar, leading to a crash afterwards.

Processed pasta and breads (otherwise known as "white" pasta or breads) are refined. They're stripped of parts of the grain when they're produced, so some vitamins and minerals are lost in the process. Some are whole foods, and others are used as ingredients in baked goods. Although we've spoken about avoiding baked goods above, if you bake your own using these ingredients, you should be good to go. Eat these in moderation, though: they're high in calories, and it can be easy to eat too much.

Healthy grains include:

- Raw oats
- Quinoa
- Barley
- Brown rice
- Bulgar wheat
- Millet
- Buckwheat
- Popcorn

Red Wine

If you need a little something, a glass of red wine a day is acceptable. While alcohol is known to be high in sugar, you may be surprised to learn that red wine contains less than a gram of sugar per 5-ounce glass. The health benefits of red wine are widely known and include lowered blood pressure, an improved cardiovascular system function, and a reduced chance of diabetes (Snopek et al., 2018).

Raw Honey

If you really can't do without sweetened coffee or adding something to your oats in the morning to sweeten them up, try raw honey. It's packed with antioxidants and has antibacterial and antifungal properties, along with a natural sweetness. Regular honey is healthier than sugar, too. Although it undergoes a pasteurization process, it's much less refined than sugar and has antibiotic properties that contribute to a healthy immune system.

How to Plan a Sugar Detox Meal

Now that you're fueled up on some knowledge about what you can and can't eat, let's get into preparation in a little more detail. Sugar detoxing is all about eating and drinking the right stuff, but you can't expect that to just fall into place—you need to do some prep work up front to make it run smoothly.

Calculating Your Sugar Intake

Although the average sugar intake fluctuates, studies have suggested that the average person consumes between 19 and 22 teaspoons of sugar every day. The American Heart Association (2018) recommends eating 9 teaspoons of added sugar per day for men (37.5 grams), and 6 teaspoons for women (25 grams). The US Dietary Guidelines recommend sticking to below 10% of your daily calorie intake in sugars.

If you wish to stick to those figures, then it's a simple case of reading every food label and making sure your daily sugar intake doesn't go over 25 grams for women and 37.5 grams for men. If you're a calorie counter, here's how you calculate how many teaspoons you should be eating:

Calculate 10% of your daily calories. For example, my daily calorie intake is 1200. 10% of that is 120. Divide that by four to get the amount in grams. As you can see, I should be eating 30 grams of sugar per day.

Divide it by four again to get teaspoons. I should be eating seven teaspoons of sugar per day at the maximum.

How to Split Your Sugar Between Meals

Since your sugar intake will fluctuate througout the day, it is important to consider your meals in advance and create some sort of meal plan. If your main meal of the day is dinner, and it's a lean protein with some vegetables and perhaps grains, your sugar levels should be down.

Make sure you avoid sauces and cook with spices for some flavor. Calculate the sugar content of each item you place on the plate. This will leave you with a certain amount of sugar to split between breakfast, lunch, and snacks. Choose your breakfast, lunch, and snack foods to fit into your sugar limit. It only takes a few weeks of doing this before you get a perfect idea of how much sugar is in various foods and can mix and match less stringently.

5-Day Sugar Detox Meal Plan

Detoxing can be a big thing. Ultimately, the end result we want is to live a life with less added sugar (or no added sugar). Five days, alone, isn't enough to build this kind of habit, but it's a start. It's just enough time not to be overwhelmed by planning and preparing meals or by trying to commit to it sternly and determinedly. That's why we're beginning with a 5-day Sugar Detox Meal Plan.

Feel free to tweak the following recipes to suit you, as long as you don't add sugar! Remember, these meals should fit into your daily calorie count, so adapt them as you need to. I will cover ideas for breakfast, lunch, dinner, snacks, and dessert. I recommend avoiding all condiments during the detox. You can cook with spices, but avoid anything that comes out of a bottle unless it's specifically sugar-free.

Spices & Sugar-Free Substitutes

If you aren't sure about cooking without your usual sauces and packet mixes, the good news is that there are plenty of spices out there that can add a ton of flavor to your food. Natural spices are okay when it comes to cooking. If you're cooking savory, there's really no point in adding sugar. If you want a tasty, flavorful meal that makes you forget about your sweet cravings, try adding the following:

- Himalayan salt
- Black pepper
- Ginger
- Turmeric (be careful: it makes everything yellow!)
- Cardamom
- Cayenne pepper
- Paprika

If you need your sweet fix, you can try adding these to desserts or even your coffee:

- Cinnamon (ground or a whole stick)
- Vanilla (extract or a whole pod)
- Nutmeg (this can be sweet or savoury)

Spices are easier to add, but fresh spice is always better! You can always add grated ginger or turmeric instead of a spice, and don't forget herbs like parsley, thyme and basic. Always double check mixed spices. Manufacturers can sometimes sneak sugar in there, and you'd never think to check the label on something like garlic salt.

If you really can't do without sweetness in your life and you need a sugar alternative that's not honey, stevia or monk fruit are natural and the healthiest of the lot. They're both extremely sweet, though, so follow serving instructions closely.

Day 1

- **Breakfast:** Omelette with stir-fry veggies (no cheese)
- **Lunch:** A salad consisting of lettuce, tomato, olives, celery, apple pieces, yellow pepper, carrots, and optional grilled chicken pieces
- **Dinner:** Zucchini spiral "pasta" with spices, mushrooms, spinach, and broccoli
- **Snack:** A handful of nuts
- **Dessert:** Plain, full-fat, unsweetened yogurt with berries

Day 2

- **Breakfast:** Oats, a drizzle of honey, and some berries
- **Lunch:** Leftover meat and veggies in a lettuce leaf "wrap"
- **Dinner:** Fish of your choice on a bed of cauliflower rice with tomato and mushrooms
- **Snack:** Two hard-boiled eggs
- **Dessert:** Sugar-free coconut water and frozen fruit popsicle (low-sugar fruit only)

Day 3

- **Breakfast:** Fruit and veggie smoothie (try it with some sugar-free peanut butter!)
- **Lunch:** Leftover cauliflower rice with cherry tomatoes, mushrooms, and peppers

- **Dinner:** Spaghetti squash and grilled, spiced chicken pieces

- **Snack:** Raw veggies and full-fat, sugar-free yogurt dip/hummus

- **Dessert:** Mixed berries "fruit salad"

Day 4

- **Breakfast:** Berries of your choice and full-fat, sugar-free yogurt

- **Lunch:** Leftover chicken pieces in a salad

- **Dinner:** Whole wheat pasta with a tomato-based sauce (sugar-free, preferably homemade)

- **Snack:** Nuts or edamame

- **Dessert:** Fruit salad (low-sugar fruits only)

Day 5

- **Breakfast:** Scrambled eggs, yellow peppers, mushrooms, & spinach (no cheese)

- **Lunch:** Vegetable salad with lettuce, spinach, broccoli, zucchini, cashews, cherry tomatoes, and olives

- **Dinner:** Homemade soup packed with low-sugar vegetables

- **Snack:** Apple slices and sugar-free peanut butter

- **Dessert:** Baked pear with walnuts and drizzled with honey

7-Day Sugar Detox Meal Plan

If you've made it through the 5-day Sugar Detox Meal Plan, congrats! It's a great first step. If you're feeling up to a slightly longer detox, here's a 7-day plan.

Day 1

- **Breakfast:** Oats, a drizzle of honey, some nuts, and some berries

- **Lunch:** Homemade soup packed with low-sugar veggies

- **Dinner:** Ginger-spiced chicken breast on cauliflower rice with broccoli pieces

- **Snack:** Raw carrot and celery sticks and full-fat, sugar-free yogurt dip/hummus (preferably homemade)

- **Dessert:** Frozen banana ice cream (blend a frozen banana in the blender until it's creamy and smooth)

Day 2

- **Breakfast:** Mix 'n Match smoothie with low-sugar fruit and veggies of your choice

- **Lunch:** Leftover chicken, shredded and added to a simple salad

- **Dinner:** Fish of your choice with salad or grilled vegetables

- **Snack:** Nuts or edamame

- **Dessert:** Apple slices and sugar-free peanut butter

Day 3

- **Breakfast:** Whole wheat toast with sugar-free peanut butter (or a sugar-free topping of your choice)

- **Lunch:** Turkey "burger" in a lettuce leaf with a slice of tomato

- **Dinner:** Zucchini/cauliflower spiral "pasta" with spiced beef strips, mushrooms, zucchini, and cherry tomatoes

- **Snack:** A handful of nuts

- **Dessert:** Sugar-free coconut water and frozen fruit popsicle

Day 4

- **Breakfast:** Oats, a drizzle of honey, and some berries

- **Lunch:** A salad consisting of lettuce, tomato, olives, celery, apple pieces, carrots, and optional grilled chicken pieces

- **Dinner:** Spiced, grilled chicken breast on a bed of cauliflower rice, roasted cabbage, and Brussels sprouts

- **Snack:** Two hard-boiled eggs

- **Dessert:** Baked pear with walnuts, drizzled with honey

Day 5

- **Breakfast:** Mix 'n Match smoothie with low-sugar fruit and veggies of your choice

- **Lunch:** Leftover chicken pieces in a salad

- **Dinner:** Your choice of fish, rice, and stir-fried vegetables

- **Snacks:** Raw veggies and full-fat, sugar-free yogurt dip/hummus

- **Dessert:** Fresh "trail mix" of berries and nuts

Day 6

- **Breakfast:** Omelette with mushrooms, spinach, and whatever other low-sugar veggies you like

- **Lunch:** Overnight oats of your choice

- **Dinner:** Meatballs and zucchini spaghetti

- **Snack:** Two hard-boiled eggs

- **Dessert:** Fruit salad (low-sugar fruit only)

Day 7

- **Breakfast:** Oats, a drizzle of honey, a handful of nuts, and some berries

- **Lunch:** Scrambled eggs on whole wheat toast

- **Dinner:** Your choice of whole wheat pasta with chicken, mushrooms, and a tomato-based, sugar-free sauce

- **Snack:** Apple slices and sugar-free peanut butter

- **Dessert:** Frozen banana ice cream and a square of sugar-free dark chocolate

Doing a quick one-week sugar detox isn't as hard as you may think it is. In fact, it's something I highly recommend doing on a regular basis if you aren't going to take a step toward becoming sugar-free permanently. Yes, it will require preparation. Yes, it will require discipline. And yes, you are going to want that sugar. However, if you can push through, satisfy your cravings with healthy foods, and begin to understand how easy it is to still eat delicious foods without needing to add sugar, you're just an arm's length away from improving your health drastically with a full sugar-free diet.

Be strong, hold your resolve, and push through when you start to fade. It'll be worth it when you start to feel more energetic, less sluggish, and realize how such a tiny, grainy molecule has been holding you back!

Key Takeaways From This Chapter

I know I have said a lot of things in this chapter but there are some key concepts that you should remember:

- Take your time with your sugar detox plan. Don't rush to get rid of your sugar cravings at once. Work more on reducing your sugar intake day by day.

- You have to be dedicated to your sugar detox program.

- Replace your sugar with other healthy food items gradually.

- Having bad sugar in your body will damage your body and life.

- Failing at one or two attempts at detoxing doesn't make you a failure. Falling short of completing your detox program isn't what matters as much as having a go at it again and until you get it right!

4. SUGAR BURNING WORKOUTS

Going on a sugar detox is not always easy. You have to be ready for the changes that your body will undergo due to the reduced amounts of sugar you now consume. In this chapter, you will discover how your body reacts to a sugar detox and how physical fitness contributes to the process. Most people are not aware of the adjustments their body has to make when they cut out sugar. They are startled by how different their body feels and may have a hard time adapting to it.

Physical fitness and exercise are very beneficial and a helpful way of tackling the fatigue and low energy that comes with cutting your sugar intake. There are various exercises that you can fit into your schedule that will help boost your energy levels, keep you fit and help you burn sugar faster while you detox. This chapter covers these exercises, including workouts that can be done while you are on the go.

The Role of Physical Fitness During A Detox

Regular exercises are very beneficial to anyone who is embarking on a sugar detox. Aside from helping you burn fat quicker and developing a more trim body, exercises will also help combat the muscle aches and pains that come with a significant reduction in sugar intake. When done correctly, you will feel stronger and more energized.

The elimination or reduction of sugar will cause a slow decline in your body's fat storage. What this means is that your body no longer has an excess supply of sugar like it did when you consumed it, thereby forcing your body to burn the extra fat for energy. This natural fat burning process takes time but when you combine a regular workout routine, especially one that features high intensity and cardio exercises with a reduced intake of sugar, you will lose significant weight much faster.

The Best Sugar Detox Exercises

It is important to create a routine that is suited to your schedule and works with your lifestyle. Many times, people make the mistake of creating elaborate routines that they do not actually follow. When trying to burn sugar, you should focus on lower intensity and endurance workouts. These include aerobic activities that help you burn off sugar that is stored in your muscles, resulting in the replacement of glycogen by the excess fat in your body.

Most people incorrectly engage in high-intensity workouts, while cutting out sugar. This can result in burnouts, dizziness, nausea, and fainting because HIIT (high-intensity interval training) requires glucose as fuel. This glucose is supplied by sugar and a combination of low glycogen levels with high-intensity exercises that results in the body breaking down muscle to burn protein for energy.

The way the body reacts to sugar burning exercises is always different from fat burning exercises. When you carry out sugar burning exercises, you become hungry, tired, and irritable after a few eating hours. This happens because sugar burners consume high carbohydrate-containing foods that elevate the blood sugar content, triggering insulin release to stabilize the blood sugar. The problem comes when the insulin brings down the blood sugar drastically, causing one to crave more sugar or carbohydrates— necessitating one to consume more sugar to keep energy in check and continuing the vicious cycle. This is why people fighting sugar addiction while exercising are always hungry and often feel tired, irritable, and cranky.

Workouts that are low intensity are more ideal and effective when it comes to burning sugar. Some of these exercises include:

- Brisk Walking
- Cycling
- Swimming
- Running
- Jogging
- Rowing
- Jumping jacks
- Yoga
- Crunches
- Pushups

15-minute workout

Most people believe they need to set aside at least an hour before they can get in a substantial workout. The truth is, however, that a 15-minute workout is effective enough to reap the physical and mental benefits during a sugar detox. Short consistent workouts are more effective than high intensity exercises done erratically. They are also very flexible and not as tasking as longer workouts.

Ideally, you should go over your schedule for the day or week and find the most convenient 15-minute blocks you can set aside for your workout. You can regulate the intensity of your workouts based on how you expect your week to go. If you are going on a long trip, you might want to replace exercises like jogging or running with yoga. For busy weeks, you can try speeding up your run or walk to give yourself a much-needed boost.

Before working out, take 1 to 3 minutes to warm up. This helps to kickstart your body and aids in circulation. Start off slow and take 2 to 4 breaks, about 30 seconds for each break. It is very easy to get carried away and over-exercise, but you must remember that when working out on a sugar detox, you can become easily exhausted due to the lack of sugar in your system.

Your main workouts should consist of two to five different exercises, each containing around two reps. When going on a walk or a run, you may be unable to include other exercises so try to maintain the same pace in order to reap the full benefits of the exercise. A 15-minute workout plan should look like this:

- 2 minutes – warm-up (jumping jacks, high knees and one spot jogging)
- 3 minutes – first set (skipping, crunches, squats and pushups)
- 30 seconds – first rest
- 3 minutes – first rep
- 30 seconds – second rest
- 3 minutes – second rep
- 30 seconds – rest
- 2 minutes – stretches (lunges and forward fold)

30-minute workout

Surprisingly, 30-minute workouts are not as fast-paced as 15-minute workouts. A lot of trainers believe that the ideal time for workouts should be half an hour. This is because 30-minute workouts allow you to fit in more exercises, take longer breaks, and are not strenuous enough to render you exhausted for the rest of the day. When running or jogging, you can go slower and pace yourself without having to watch the clock as you would on a shorter workout. 30-minute workouts are perfect for cultivating a healthy lifestyle and are proven to boost your mood.

A 30-minute workout plan should look like this:

- 4 minutes – warm-up (jumping jacks, high knees, one spot jogging)
- 7 minutes – first set (skipping, crunches, squats, pushups)
- 30 seconds – first rest
- 7 minutes – first rep
- 30 seconds – second rest
- 7 minutes – second rep
- 1 minute – rest
- 3 minutes – stretches (lunges, forward fold, yoga)

90-minute workout

Workouts such as cycling, swimming, rowing, running, hiking, and other outdoor exercises are best suited for this duration. Typically, workouts that last this long are very low in intensity and are usually done on days with an empty schedule. Keeping a steady pace helps to kickstart weight loss and increase the flow of blood.   This type of workout is also considered low risk, with less strain on the knees and other joints, reducing the occurrence of injury.

Even though you do not emerge from a steady, low intensity workout coated in sweat, sugar is still burnt. Most low intensity exercises done for extended periods of time are easy to do and are adaptable to your circumstance.

The Best Exercises While On the Go

Many times, people find it difficult to maintain an exercise routine because they are away from the gym or do not have the appropriate machines to work with. When they do return home, it feels like a struggle to start all over because of how much progress they lost when traveling or on the go.

Hiking, cycling and other outdoor activities are a great way to get some exercise while on vacation. The best part about these activities is they do not feel like working out because you spend time exploring. There are many exercises that require minimal space and no equipment that can be done on the go. Travel workouts go a long way in boosting your energy as you continue your sugar detox, helping you avoid relapses in your sugar consumption. Some exercises you can squeeze in while on the go include:

- Jumping jacks
- Pushups (e.g. elevated pushups)
- Lunges (e.g. walking lunges, assisted lunges)
- Planks
- Squats (e.g. bodyweight squats)

How To Optimize Your Sugar Detox Workout

Sugar burns quickly in comparison to fat and leaves behind lactic acid. You can store between 200 – 400 grams of sugar in your muscles, depending on how much lean muscle you have on your frame. Once your frame has reached its limit in sugar storage, it begins to convert any excess sugar consumed to fat. When you begin exercising during a sugar detox, you have to remember to take it slow and not put too much pressure on yourself. A change in eating patterns ultimately requires a change in exercise.

Exercise is very beneficial as it improves metabolism, and stimulates elimination channels such as the skin (through sweat) and the lungs (through the breath). Here are some things to remember while working out during a sugar detox:

1. Exercise for shorter durations

When you are on a sugar detox, your body is short on fuel to carry you through longer periods of exercise. If your workout routine is intense, try as much as possible to reduce the duration so that you do not push yourself to exhaustion. A run, for example, is higher in intensity than a walk and should take less time. It is very important to keep your workouts within the 30-minute range particularly if you are consuming fiber to aid digestion, since fiber is a poor source of energy to sustain you during workouts.

2. Reduce the intensity of your workouts

It is essential that you cut down the intensity of your workouts when on a detox diet. The sugars and carbohydrates in your diet supply your blood with glucose, which in turn provides the fuel required for intense workouts. While on a sugar detox, you might feel dizzy or faint during exercises so try to cut out high-intensity exercises and stick to workouts that are paced moderately and not strenuous to complete.

3. Do exercises that are lower impact

To reduce how much stress you put on your body while working out during a detox, reduce the impact of your exercises. A good example is a brisk walk, which helps you maintain necessary levels of fitness as you detoxify your body. Due to your restrictive diet, you may experience fatigue if you take on high-intensity exercises.

4. Do stretching exercises

A low impact method of keeping your muscles active is by enganging in flexibility boosting exercises. These can include yoga, Tai Chi, or stretch classes. It is important to target the major muscle groups located in your arms, legs, and back. The more agile you are, the more sugar you burn.

5. Listen to your body and do not overwork yourself

When exercising in line with your detox diet, the key is to make sure you work within your limits. Take note of how your body reacts to every workout and be ready to stop at the first sign of fatigue. Remember to remain hydrated and consume more protein to prevent muscle loss. On days you feel stronger or are very motivated to exercise, do not be scared to keep going for a bit longer than usual.

Key Takeaways

In this chapter, we have discussed the effects of sugar detoxing on the human body and the importance of exercise in dieting. Here are the most important points to note from this chapter:

- A sugar detox will make you lose weight but you will experience faster and more significant changes if you include exercises.
- While on a detox, your body's energy levels are low, so try to avoid high-intensity workouts.
- In order to avoid fatigue or burnouts, make sure you take it slow when you begin working out while dieting.

In the next chapter, you will discover how to handle the cravings that come with sugar detoxing and how to tackle withdrawal symptoms when maintaining a zero-sugar lifestyle.

5. Maintaining a Zero Sugar Lifestyle

Without question, there are certain principles to know when you want to cut down your sugar consumption and maintain an overall healthy lifestyle. This chapter is dedicated to the best practices to ensure you stay on course with your zero sugar diet.

The 7 Key Principles To Maintain a Zero Sugar Diet

1. **Start Slowly**

When you want to start the zero sugar diet, it is normal to be full of enthusiasm because you started a new, worthwhile pursuit. However, you should begin gradually and slowly. You must create an eating plan that you can follow easily. You should not eliminate sugar entirely from your diet at the beginning of this process, as it would be difficult to follow. Start with cutting down your sugar consumption for the first few weeks. This allows your body to adjust to lower sugar levels and reduce cravings. At this early stage, it is normal to experience sugar withdrawal symptoms. Later in this chapter, I will discuss the most effective ways to deal with these symptoms.

Quick Tips
   a. Replace soda with natural fruit juices containing no added sugars.

b. Make sure any bread with your meals does not contain added sugars.

c. Reduce the amount of supplemental sugar you add in your beverages and cereals.

d. Settle for plain, unflavored yogurts rather than the fully flavored ones.

2. Stay away from sugary desserts.

It should come as no surprise that most desserts contain a high level of added sugar. This, of course, includes cake, ice cream, cookies, and muffins. It is important to accept that these foods are the enemy of a sugar detox and should be avoided at all costs.

3. Check labels of all foods you buy.

As discussed in the previous chapters, certain types of foods have "hidden" sugars that fall under different names, as discussed earlier in this book. Pay careful attention to items like beans, bread, pasta, rice, crackers and tacos.

Reminder

- 4 grams of sugar is equal to one teaspoon

4. Stay away from artificial sweeteners.

Artificial sweeteners are usually sweeter than sugar. Consuming them only makes your brain think you are eating sugar, thereby causing you to crave sugar more.

5. Monitor what you drink.

When you embark on a zero sugar diet, it is important to monitor everything you are drinking. Stay away from soda, hot chocolate, flavored coffee, flavored tea, wine and cocktails. You can substitute these drinks by infusing water with fruits or making smoothies with unflavored yogurt.

6. **Use more flavor instead of sugar.**

A zero sugar diet does not mean you should consume bland foods. Feel free to use flavor, seasoning and other spices to make your meals taste great. For example, you can use vanilla for meals you would otherwise use sugar with. You can also use added spice like cinnamon or pumpkin spice for your unflavored yogurts.

7. **Total abstinence is not necessary.**

As much as you want to cut down or eliminate sugar from your diet, it will not be easy. Indeed, there will be days when you want to eat cake or indulge in some ice cream. It is important to remember you can still consume the recommended daily allowance of sugar. Men can take up to nine teaspoons of sugar a day and women can consume six teaspoons of daily sugar.

How to Fight Sugar Cravings

When you decide to cut down on your sugar intake, there are going to be times when you are unable to hold back your cravings, so it is essential to know how to curb and manage them. Before jumping straight into the management of cravings, I first want to discuss why they occur in the first place.

Why Do We Crave Sugar?

If you have sugar cravings, it is important to understand that they are normal. The cravings we have for sugary foods and carbohydrates are motivated by the need to improve our mood, since sugary treats increase the levels of serotonin in the brain. The role serotonin plays in our body system is to boost our sense of well-being. As mentioned earlier, it is a feel-good hormone. Here are the most common reasons why we crave sugary treats:

1. **Physical and Emotional Stress**

"Stress-eating" is an eating pattern that most often occurs when people experience stress in their relationships, work, school and home. Sugary foods are usually the food of choice when one feels down and needs to feel lifted up.

2. **Sleep Deprivation**

Sleep deprivation also leads to an increase in stress levels, which inevitably leads to the stress-eating pattern. Cravings then increase for sugary treats, carbohydrates and salty foods. Studies have shown that we tend to make poor decisions regarding what we eat or drink when tired.

3. **Nutrient Imbalance**

Some people do not pay close attention to what they eat and wonder why they get hungry after a short period of time. If you eat a meal low in protein, fiber or healthy fats you will feel hungry again shortly after. Inevitably, our bodies will then crave sugary treats when low on energy.

4. **Low Calorie Diet**

There is usually an intense craving for sugar in individuals who fast or do not have time to eat well. This intense sugar craving is owed to the fact that the body is low on energy, and this is when the body craves sugar the most.

5. **Deficiency of Micronutrients**

There is evidence that a deficiency in magnesium may lead to increased sugar cravings. According to various studies, some individuals might experience an increased desire for sugar, which might be due to magnesium deficiency.

How They Compare: Cravings vs. Addiction

Most individuals do not understand the difference between sugar cravings and sugar addiction. There are counter studies with one side suggesting that sugar is not addictive, while the other side indicates that it is. Since there is much confusion in the medical world, it is necessary to understand the difference between both.

Addiction is said to happen when there is a strong need or compulsion to consume a substance. This compulsion then leads to an uncontrollable use, where stopping would lead to physical withdrawal symptoms. In the case of sugar, some individuals experience withdrawal symptoms when they decide to cut it out of their diet. The overall addiction to sugar is owed to individual dependence on how it makes them feel when they consume it. In sugar addiction management, trained professionals like a nutritionist or a dietician are usually required. Sugar cravings, however, can be dealt with on your own.

To keep it simple, if you experience withdrawal symptoms when you halt sugar consumption, you have an addiction.

6 Key Habits That Fight Cravings

As stated earlier, you can deal with sugar cravings on your own. Fighting your cravings might not be easy at first, but trust in the process. It is essential to understand that your body will need time to adjust to a zero sugar diet. The following tips are practical ways to help prevent any initial cravings that might arise.

1. **Use artificial sweeteners with caution**

Artificial sweeteners can be healthy in terms of its benefits in cutting calories, but at the same time, they are unhealthy when trying to cut your overall sugar intake. As much as these sweeteners help reduce calories, the unfortunate side effect of overconsuming these sweeteners is an increase in sugar cravings.

2. Get enough nutrients

If you are unaware of daily intake of nutrients, you may need the help of a registered dietician to help ensure you have the right eating plan that would give you the macronutrients and micronutrients you need. As stated earlier, magnesium deficiency can lead to an increase in sugar cravings. You can acquire magnesium from nuts, seeds and whole grains.

3. Make sure to get enough sleep

One of the leading causes of high sugar consumption is the lack of adequate sleep. Getting enough sleep is very important to living healthy. If you get enough sleep, you will have enough energy and your body will not crave sugar for sustained daily energy.

4. Eat healthy carbohydrates

Studies suggest that we gain 45% to 65% of daily calories from carbohydrates. This means that for every 2,000 calories per day, we acquire about 1,300 calories from carbs. You can acquire healthy carbohydrates from fruits, whole grains and vegetables. Sweeter vegetables like sweet potatoes and sweet corn are a great substitute for sugar cravings.

5. Use more raw fruits

Early cravings can also be dealt with by consuming raw fruits such as berries, oranges, bananas and melons to provide the sweetness you crave together with other benefits like high fiber and vitamins.

Tips to stock up your kitchen

- Get enough fruits. When you get sugar cravings, fruits will serve as an appropriate alternative rather than sugary treats.

- Get protein-rich foods and fiber-rich foods such as plain yogurt, unsweetened oatmeal and eggs.

- Drink enough water. At the early stages of cutting sugar intake, you should reduce consumption of soda and sweetened coffee and tea drinks.

- Consider chewing sugar-free gum to serve as an alternative to dealing with sugar cravings.

6. Get support

It will be challenging at the beginning to cut back on sugar consumption, so you will need to seek as much support as you can from fellow dieters, friends, and family.

Without a doubt, having people around you who can give you the support and motivation you need, will help you immensely on this new journey.

Identifying Symptoms of Sugar Withdrawal

Some individuals are not aware of the symptoms associated with sugar withdrawal, and people who know about it are scared of the signs. Because of this, they are reluctant to go on a detox. As stated earlier, withdrawal symptoms are experienced by people with a sugar addiction. It is important to note that these symptoms are temporary and can be managed. Before discussing the ways to manage these symptoms, it is important that each symptom be highlighted. When you decide to quit sugar consumption, you might experience all or some of the following conditions:

1. Cravings

Cravings are the most common symptom of sugar withdrawal, and it can also be challenging to manage. Cravings can be terrible, and sometimes individuals who experience this often fall back into heavy sugar consumption. The management of this symptom will be discussed in the next section.

2. Mood Swings

Some individuals may experience mood swings. They are easily irritated and cranky, and this is because they do not get the feel-good emotions that sugar gives them. This makes them feel anxious, and they have to go back to the massive consumption of sugar. However, this goes away after some time.

3. Depression

Depression is not common, but some individuals may experience it. This is due to the lower levels of serotonin secretion. Since sugar is said to increase serotonin's secretion, which gives the feel-good feeling, cutting down its consumption may lead to depression in specific individuals.

4. Fatigue

Sugar gives an energy boost when consumed, and this provides the "feel-good" emotion. Cutting sugar consumption means you won't get the energy added sugar gives you, and therefore may experience fatigue.

5. Sleep Irregularities

One of the symptoms experienced when the consumption of sugar is reduced is irregularity in sleep. Some individuals experience this symptom, and it is due to changes in blood sugar levels and anxiety.

6. **Headaches**

Most individuals experience headaches, which are caused by changes in body chemistry. When the body is used to a high level of sugar, cutting it from your daily diet forces the body to adjust to this change. During this adjustment, some people experience disruptive symptoms like headaches.

7. **Muscle Aches and Tremors**

Muscle aches and cramps can be experienced by some individuals, however, it is not a common symptom of sugar withdrawal. Another uncommon symptom is body tremors.

Managing Sugar Withdrawal Symptoms

In the management of sugar withdrawal symptom, the main aim is to avoid hunger. Getting hungry triggers your body's craving for sugar. If it does not get the amount of sugar it needs, then the withdrawal symptoms start to kick in. In order not to stay hungry, add proteins, fruits, fibers, and sweet substitutes to your meal plan. Foods with all these are healthy and will help you through the journey of living the zero sugar diet. For the headaches and pains, a pain reliever can be used to get rid of them, and in some cases, they wear off without using medications.

Remember, you are improving your health by quitting high sugar consumption, so focus on the bigger picture, and always remember that these symptoms are temporary.

6. Sugar Replacements

The best way to cut out sugar in your diet is to do it gradually. This will not only help you transition to alternative food options, but it will also help your body slowly adjust, potentially cutting out withdrawal symptoms.

As you begin to cut out sugar from your diet, look to replace it with alternatives that are going to give your body what it needs. Look to healthy fats like nuts, avocados, cheese, dark chocolate, and whole eggs. Ramp up your intake of leafy greens. Eat clean proteins like beans, grains, nuts, and seeds. Replace refined sugar with healthy sugars found in berries and other fruits. Finally, make sure that you drink plenty of water. Water is key to keeping your body healthy as you detox from sugar. Remember that the commonly suggested water intake is eight, 8-ounce cups of water per day.

The following is a list of foods to help you curb your sugar cravings.

1. Dark Chocolate

The most sought after choice of food for people craving sugary treats is chocolate. As an alternative, you can consume a healthier choice of chocolate by going for dark chocolates. Dark chocolates contain polyphenols, which have anti-inflammatory and antioxidant properties beneficial to your health. Dark chocolates, however, also contain a small amount of added sugar, you should also consume with caution and monitor your recommended daily allowance of sugar.

2. Chia Seeds

The chia seed is a nutritious food that contains some beneficial nutrients like soluble dietary fiber and omega-3 fatty acids. The soluble fiber absorbs water and swells up in your gut, making you feel full. This, in turn, prevents you from having sugar cravings. Another good thing about chia seeds is that they can satisfy your sweet cravings if you make them into the chia pudding.

3. Sugar-free Gum and Mints

Sugar-free gums and mints contain artificial sweeteners with low calories and no added sugar. Gums and mints are very effective in controlling cravings, hunger, and binge eating.

4. Sweet Potatoes

Sweet potatoes, as the name implies, are sweet and filling. They are a source of carbohydrates, as well as, vitamins, minerals, and fiber. Sweet potatoes can fill you up and also give you the sweet taste you need when cravings strike.

5. Medjool Dates

Medjool dates are sweet, dry fruits that are very nutritious. They contain fiber, iron, and potassium. Medjool dates are also a perfect substitute for candy and soda when you crave sugary treats. You can even create a healthy, sweet snack when combining dates with nuts.

6. Yogurt

Yogurts are very nutritious and high in protein. They might not be able to give you the sweet sensation you crave, but they can help control your hunger and heavy enough to fill you up.

7. Smoothies

Smoothies are a blended mixture of various fruits with yogurt as an additive. They are delightful and nutritious, while also filling. If you need something sweet and filling in place of chocolates, candy, soda; you can settle for smoothies. To leverage the full benefits of smoothies, use with raw, whole fruit.

8. Sugar-free Beverages

It's no secret that beverages like soda contain high amounts and sugar and sweeteners. Since it can be difficult for those just starting a detox to cut out soda completely, you should settle for sugar-free beverages, which is equally sweet but without sugar and calories. It is advised to drink with caution.

9. Eggs

Eggs contain a high amount of protein, and it helps to control appetite and overall food cravings. When eggs are consumed, they suppress the hunger hormone ghrelin. It is advised to have eggs for breakfast, so you remain full for most of the day.

10. Whole Grains

Whole grains contain beneficial nutrients like iron, phosphorus, magnesium, vitamins, manganese, and selenium. They are also high in fiber, which provides a feeling of fullness and therefore regulates hunger and cravings. Whole fibers also help regulate the gut by allowing the growth of beneficial bacteria.

Meal Planning with Substitutes

When you make a meal plan, you can visualize where you normally consume the most sugar and pragmatically replace them with healthy options. Here are some meal suggestions to give you a visualization of what your daily meals can look like.

Breakfast

Breakfast is actually quite easy to find alternatives to sugary foods. Of course, cut out processed cereals and pastries, and opt for more proteins and healthy fats to jump start your day. Example breakfast meals include:

- Oatmeal
- Basically any egg dish like boiled or scrambled eggs, or a delectable omelet that includes peppers or leafy greens to liven it up
- Fiber-based cereal. Consider adding nuts like almonds or berries
- Be conscious of any sugar added to your morning tea or coffee (also watch what types of juice you consume in the early hours)
- Smoothie made with berries, oatmeal, nuts, and skim milk

Lunch

For lunch, keep the clean proteins coming, and mix in some leafy greens to not only add color to your plate, but also to keep you energized throughout the day.

- Chicken stir-fry with veggies
- Tuna salad
- Vegetable curry with a side of rice
- Low-fat burger that's grilled, not fried (try a turkey or veggie patty)
- Chicken tortilla or veggie wrap
- Salad with nuts, berries, and chicken

Dinner

For dinner, you want to have a healthy amount of carbs to sustain you throughout the evening and into the next morning. We don't want any midnight sugar binges because we didn't eat enough at dinner.

- Whole wheat pasta with tomato or vegetable sauce. Add some cheeses like parmesan for added healthy fat
- Vegetable pizza with a side salad
- Grilled fillet steak with baked sweet potato, mushrooms, and tomatoes
- Hearty chilli with different types of beans and chicken or lean beef as added protein

Sugar Free Desserts and Snacks

Here are a few quick and easy recipes for desserts and snacks that are so good that will trick your sweet tooth into thinking that they are filled with sugar.

Chocolate Fudge

Ingredients:

- 2 packages of cream cheese (8 oz each), softened
- 2 oz unsweetened chocolate, melted and cooled to room temperature
- 1 tsp stevia or sugar substitute equivalent to one cup of sugar
- 1 tsp vanilla extract
- ½ cup of chopped pecans or preferred nuts

Directions:

1. In a small bowl, beat ingredients until smooth. Stir in nuts.
2. Press into a lined 8-inch baking dish.
3. Cover and refrigerate overnight. Keep chilled.

Notes:

- This recipe has a higher amount of dairy so it should be stored in the fridge.
- You can make this dairy-free by substituting the cream cheese for a vegan cream-cheese alternative.
- Looking to try something new? Consider swapping out the chopped nuts for dried fruit or swap out the vanilla extract

for a different flavor. Looking for a little kick? Sprinkle a small amount of chilli pepper on top.

Sugar-Free Apple Pie

Ingredients:

- 1 tsp stevia or sugar substitute equivalent to one cup of sugar
- ¼ cup cornstarch
- 1 tsp cinnamon
- Pastry for double-crust pie
- 8 cups of thinly sliced apples (your choice)
- 1 tbsp butter, melted

Directions:

1. In a large bowl, combine the first three ingredients.
2. Fold the apples into the mixture.
3. Line the pie pan with the bottom crust.
4. Add apples to the pan. Brush with butter.
5. Roll out the remaining pie crust over the top of the filling. Add slits to the top. Seal edges.
6. Bake at 375-degrees F for 35 minutes. Then increase the oven temperature to 400-degrees F for another 15-20 minutes.

Notes:

- You can use any sugar substitute for this recipe. To keep the grainy texture of normal sugar by using stevia or coconut sugar.

Sugar-Free Chocolate Chip Cookies

Ingredients:

-
- 2 ¼ cup flour
- 1 tsp baking soda
- 1 cup + 1 tbsp butter, softened to room temperature
- 1 tsp stevia or 1 cup of white sugar alternative
- ½ cup of brown sugar alternative
- 2 eggs
- 1 tsp vanilla extract
- Sugar-free chocolate chips

Directions:

1. Preheat the oven to 350 degrees F. Prep the baking sheet with non-stick spray or with parchment paper. Opt for a zero waste alternative by using silicone baking mats.
2. In a medium bowl, combine flour and baking soda. Set aside.
3. In a mixing bowl, cream butter and sugar.
4. Add the dry ingredients to the creamed butter and sugar. For best results, combine half of the dry ingredients, mix with the butter, then add the remaining dry ingredients. Add eggs and vanilla extract.
5. Fold in chocolate chips.
6. Scoop cookies onto the baking sheet. Bake for 10-12 minutes. Larger cookies will take longer to cook.

Granola Yogurt Popsicles

Ingredients:

- 1 ⅓ cup dairy-free yogurt
- ¼ cup unsweetened coconut milk (or milk of choice)
- 2 tbsp honey
- ⅓ cup of granola
- 1 sliced kiwi (or fruit of choice)
- ¼ cup of blueberries (or fruit of choice)

Directions:

1. In a bowl whisk together yogurt, milk, and honey until smooth.
2. Drop sliced fruit (first choice) into the bottom of five popsicle molds.
3. In layers, add yogurt mixture, blueberries (or fruit of choice), then yogurt again. Leave about ¼ inch at the top.
4. Fill the remaining mold with granola. Add popsicle sticks.
5. Freeze at least 4 hours before serving.

Notes:

- There are many ways to switch this recipe up. Swap out the fruit suggestions for fun combos or choose a flavored yogurt for an extra punch of flavor.

Sugar Detox Shopping List

Most people don't realize how much of an impact sugar actually has on their day-to-day lives until they kick it to the curb. In our modern diets, sugar is everywhere. On food labels, sugar can be called more than 50 different names which means that it can hide nearly in plain sight. So how can we break free from this confusion?

Here are some easy ways to find some sugar-free food at the grocery store.

Fruits

Although the sugar in fruit is better than refined sugar, it is still best to focus on fruits that are lower in sugar when you are trying to cut sugar out of your diet. When you are in the store, look for these healthy and low-sugar fruit options.

- Lemons/limes
- Kiwi
- Raspberries
- Strawberries
- Blackberries
- Grapefruit
- Avocados
- Watermelon
- Cantaloupe/honeydew
- Oranges
- Peaches

Snacks

Processed foods are often loaded with hidden sugars, but what do you look for when you want an easy to grab snack that you don't have to prepare ahead of time? Here are some ideas for you to grab on your next trip to the store.

- Nuts. Almonds are great!
- Tortilla chips with salsa
- Dark chocolate bars
- Munchable granola (read labels, watch out for granola bars)
- Hummus or roasted chickpeas
- Quinoa chips
- Plain yogurts (flavored yogurts is where the sugar is usually added)
- Popcorn without flavoring. You can add your own healthy alternative flavoring at home

Canned Goods

Canned goods are essentials to have in your pantry to prepare your next lunch and dinner. Here are some sugar-free staples to keep stocked up on.

- Canned spinach. This is a better alternative to fresh spinach because it doesn't go bad as quickly!
- Refried black beans. Great source of protein and is perfect for taco tuesdays!
- Coconut milk
- Canned tuna
- Some canned soups. Just watch out for sodium levels in these.
- Pinto beans. These are naturally low in sodium and a great plant protein to add to your next soup or chilli.

- Pure pumpkin puree. This is a great staple to have for dessert recipes (sugar-free of course) and even soups!
- Tomato sauce. Opt for unflavored sauces that you can spice up at home.
- Corn. Great as its own side dish or added to salsas and soups.
- Beans, beans, beans. Stock up on all of the bean varieties because there are endless uses for them!

Note: Be very wary of canned fruits. Often, they are packed with added sugars (even if they say that they don't on their can). It's always best to buy fruits fresh or at least frozen. Remember that you can always freeze fresh fruits to save for later!

Conclusion

In this book, you have read a lot about how bad sugar is for your health and how you can cure sugar addiction. The zero sugar lifestyle has gained increasing popularity over the years because most people now see the importance and benefit of cutting sugar from their diet. Research has adequately shown that the reduction or complete elimination of sugar reduces the risk of having diseases like diabetes and helps prevent obesity.

Sugar detox is a way of cleansing your body system of the excess sugar you have consumed so far, and for that journey to be successful, you need to find the best foods to eat that will help in your detox journey. When you are able to map out a meal plan and stick with it, then you have succeeded in staying away from excess sugar consumption.

Before stepping out in the morning, be sure to have enough breakfast so you won't be tempted to snack on junk food because you were hungry. If it is possible, you can also prepare lunch and pack it to work or fill your bag with fruits and veggies that can stand in as your snack. Avoid eating out completely so you don't get tempted to return to sugary foods, it is healthier to eat at home. When you do all of this, you will find yourself staying further away from sugar and controlling your cravings. In fact, if you follow the steps religiously, your craving for sugar will die out. Another way of fighting your craving for sugar is to stay away from alcohol.

With this book, I have covered some useful ways in which you can break free from sugar addiction. Although, most people get addicted in various ways and their symptoms also vary, the fact is everyone who is addicted to sugar face similar struggles. Even though it might seem like a simple task to cut sugar from your daily meal plan, some barriers usually pop up just in time to prevent you from achieving your goals.

You are advised to read this book carefully and know the damages excess sugar can do to your body and how important it is for you to stay clear from excessive added sugars. However, you need to take things slow and steady. Take your new diet one day at a time, since it is not possible for you to stop your intake of sugar all at once. You can start by reducing your daily intake of sugary meals, then gradually put an end to it.

Fear not, since there is still a chance for you to change. Once you know that you are addicted to sugar, you can easily trace where the problem is coming from and start from there to fix your addiction problem. I hope this book has been a helpful guide for you to know what addiction to sugar is, and how detrimental it is to your health.

Let today be the first step in your journey to a healthier you!

Bibliography

WebMD (2003, Nov. 14). Have A Sweet Tooth? *WebMD*. Retrived from: https://www.webmd.com/mental-health/addiction/news/20031114/have-sweet-tooth-beware-of-alcoholism

Hughes, L. (2019, Dec 17). How Does Too Much Sugar Affect Your Body? *WebMD*. Retrieved from: https://www.webmd.com/diabetes/features/how-sugar-affects-your-body

Appelo, T. (2017, Oct 10). More Proof Sugar Can Kill. *AARP*. Retrieved from: https://www.aarp.org/health/healthy-living/info-2017/health-effects-high-sugar-diet-fd.html

Hatanaka, M. (2020, June 30). What is the impact of eating too much sugar? *Medical News Today*. Retrieved from: https://www.medicalnewstoday.com/articles/eating-too-much-sugar

Seidenberg, C. (2018, Jan 30). Why do we crave sugar, and how to beat the habit ? *Washington Post*. Retrieved from: https://www.washingtonpost.com/lifestyle/wellness/explaining-the-siren-song-of-sugar-and-how-to-beat-the-habit/2018/01/26/8a9557f8-f7ae-11e7-a9e3-ab18ce41436a_story.html

Daily Sabah. (2020, Apr 15). The science behind sugar cravings: Why we crave it and how to beat it. *Daily Sabah*. Retrieved from: https://www.google.com/amp/s/www.dailysabah.com/life/health/the-science-behind-sugar-cravings-why-we-crave-it-and-how-to-beat-it/amp

Dwyer, L. (2016, Apr 13). Kicking Sugar Is as Tough as Beating a Cocaine Habit. *Take Part*. Retrieved from: http://www.takepart.com/article/2016/04/13/kicking-sugar-addiction-tough-beating-cocaine-habit

Harris & Bargh. (2009, Oct 24). The Relationship between Television viewing and Unhealthy Eating: Implications for Children and Media Interventions. *NCBI*. Retrieved from: https://www.ncbi.nlm.nih.gov/pmc/articles/PMC2829711/

The Jakarta Post. (2019, June 10). Six signs of sugar addiction. *The Jakarta Post*. Retrieved from; https://www.google.com/amp/s/www.thejakartapost.com/amp/life/2019/06/10/six-signs-of-sugar-addiction.html

Santos-Longhurst, A. (2020, Aug 20). What Is a Sugar Detox? Effects and How to Avoid Sugar. *Healthline*. Retrieved from; https://www.healthline.com/health/sugar-detox-symptoms#symptoms

Brooks, M. (2020, Apr 30). Sweet death: how the sugar industry created a global crisis. *New Statesman*. Retrieved from; https://www.newstatesman.com/culture/books/2017/01/sweet-death-how-sugar-industry-created-global-crisis

Avena, M. (2007, May 18). Evidence for sugar addiction: Behavioral and neurochemical effects of intermittent, excessive sugar intake. *NCBI*. Retrieved from; https://www.ncbi.nlm.nih.gov/pmc/articles/PMC2235907/

Choi, J. (2016). What to Expect When You

me Go On a Sugar Detox. *What Great Grand Maate*. Retrieved from;
https://whatgreatgrandmaate.com/what-to-expect-when-you-go-on-a-sugar-detox/

Coyle, D. (2020). A Beginner's Guide to the Low Glycemic Diet. *Healthline*. Retrieved from;
https://www.healthline.com/nutrition/low-glycemic-diet#factors-affecting-gi
De Medeiros, M. (2018). Your 2-Week Sugar Detox. Popsugar. Retrieved from;
https://www.popsugar.com/fitness/Two-Week-Sugar-Detox-44271478

Gunnars, K. (2016). Good Carbs, Bad Carbs— How to Make the Right Choices. *Healthline*. Retrieved from:
https://www.healthline.com/nutrition/good-carbs-bad-carbs#TOC_TITLE_HDR_4

Are You A Sugar Burner or a Fat Burning? Listen To Your Body. *Prospect Medical Systems*. (n.d.). Retrieved from:
https://www.prospectmedical.com/are-you-sugar-burner-or-fat-burning-listen-your-body-0

Bennett, B. (2014, April 13). Sugar Detox Phase 1 Week 1 Menu Plan. *Sugar-Free Mom*. Retrieved from:
https://www.sugarfreemom.com/phase-one/sugar-detox-phase-1-week-1-menu-plan/

Collins, M. (2020, February 28). 10-Day Sugar Detox Menu Plan Made Easy. *Sugar Addiction*. Retrieved from:
https://sugaraddiction.com/10-day-sugar-detox-menu-plan-made-easy/

Curp, C. (2019, October 21). Superfood Sheet Pan Omelet (Whole30, Paleo, Keto). *The Castaway Kitchen*. Retrieved from:
https://thecastawaykitchen.com/2017/12/superfood-sheet-pan-omelet-paleo-keto-whole30/

Food, F. (2020, February 19). Sugar Detox 2019 Meal Plan. *Further Food*. Retrieved from:
https://www.furtherfood.com/sugar-detox-meal-plan-2019/

McCoy, J. (2018, April 18). 10 Sugar

Cleanse-Friendly Snacks That Will Satisfy Even the Strongest Sweet Tooth. *Cooking Light*. Retrieved from:
https://www.cookinglight.com/eating-smart/nutrition-101/healthy-low-sugar-snacks

McLintock, K. (2017, December 2). 4 Sugar Detox Recipes to Help You Recover From Your Cookie Coma. *Byrdie*. Retrieved from:
https://www.byrdie.com/sugar-detox-recipes

Sanfilippo, D. (n.d.). Breakfast Archives. *21-Day Sugar Detox*. Retrieved from:
https://21daysugardetox.com/content-category/breakfast/

Blackburn, K. B. (2019, May 8). Sugar detox: Get the facts. *MD Anderson*. Retrieved from:
https://www.mdanderson.org/publications/focused-on-health/sugar-detox.h22Z1592202.html

Codella, R. (2017, December 15). Sugars, exercise, and health. *PubMed*. Retrieved from:
https://pubmed.ncbi.nlm.nih.gov/27817910/

Eske, J. (2019, October 7). What to know about sugar detox symptoms. *Medical news today*. Retrieved from:
https://www.medicalnewstoday.com/articles/326575#treatments

Laskowski, R. (2019, April 27). Exercise: How much do I need every day?. *Mayo Clinic*. Retrieved from:
https://www.mayoclinic.org/healthy-lifestyle/fitness/expert-answers/exercise/faq-20057916

Greenlaw, E. (2013, January 15). Exercises to Lower Your Blood Sugar. *WebMD*. Retrieved from:
https://www.webmd.com/healthy-aging/features/exercise-lower-blood-sugar#1

Osborn, C. (2020, January 21). How Long Does Withdrawal From Sugar Last? (n.d.). *Verywell Mind*. Retrieved from:
https://www.verywellmind.com/sugar-withdrawal-symptoms-timeline-and-treatment-4176257

L. (2019, February 27). How to Reduce Fat with High-Intensity Sugar-Burning Workout. *LivingBetter50*. Retrieved from: https://www.livingbetter50.com/reduce-fat-high-intensity-sugar-burning-workout/

Lopez, S. (2020, January 10). 10 Workouts to do While traveling *Skinny Ms*. Retrieved from: https://skinnyms.com/10-workouts-to-do-while-traveling-2/

Santos-Longhurst, A. (2020, August 20). What Is a Sugar Detox? Effects and How to Avoid Sugar. *Healthline* Retrieved from: https://www.healthline.com/health/sugar-detox-symptoms#side-effects

Warner, J. (2012, August 24). 30 Minutes of Daily Exercise Enough to Shed Pounds. *WebMD*. Retrieved from: https://www.webmd.com/fitness-exercise/news/20120824/30-minutes-daily-exercise-shed-pounds#:%7E:text=After%2013%20weeks%2C%20the%20study,worked%20out%20for%20an%20hour.

Zinczenko, D. (2019, March 8). The Greatest High-intensity Sugar-burning Workout to Cut Body Fat. *Men's Journal*. Retrieved from: https://www.mensjournal.com/health-fitness/greatest-high-intensity-sugar-burning-workout-cut-body-fat/

Cockayne, L. M. (2020, July 9). Sugar Withdrawal - All you need to know. *Make me sugar free* Retrieved from: Https://Www.Makemesugarfree.Com/Post/Sugar-Withdrawal-Everything-You-Ever-Need-to-Know.

Farey, M. (2020). How to Help Curb Sugar Cravings. *Verywell Fit*. Retrieved from: https://www.verywellfit.com/how-to-stop-sugar-cravings-quick-tips-for-relief-4174995

West, R. H. D. (2018, January 8). 19 Foods That Can Fight Sugar Cravings. *Healthline*. Retrieved from: https://www.healthline.com/nutrition/foods-that-fight-sugar-cravings#TOC_TITLE_HDR_19

Whelan, C. (2017, October 12). No-Sugar Diet: 10 Tips to Get Started. *Healthline* Retrieved from: https://www.healthline.com/health/food-nutrition/no-sugar-diet#save-it-for-special-occasions

(2019, November 5) The sweet danger of sugar. *Health Harvard*. Retrieved from: https://www.health.harvard.edu/heart-health/the-sweet-danger-of-sugar

Cantwell, M., & Elliott, C. (2017). Nitrates, Nitrites and Nitrosamines from Processed Meat Intake and ColorectalCancer Risk. *Journal of Clinical Nutrition & Dietetics*, 03(04). https://doi.org/10.4172/2472-1921.100062

How much water do you need to stay healthy? (2020, October 14). Mayo Clinic. https://www.mayoclinic.org/healthy-lifestyle/nutrition-and-healthy-eating/in-depth/water/art-20044256#:~:text=The%20U.S.%20National%20Academies%20of

Johnson, R. K., Appel, L. J., Brands, M., Howard, B. V., Lefevre, M., Lustig, R. H., Sacks, F., Steffen, L. M., & Wylie-Rosett, J. (2009). Dietary Sugars Intake and Cardiovascular Health. *Circulation*, 120(11), 1011–1020. https://doi.org/10.1161/circulationaha.109.192627

Lehman, S. (2020, December 2). *Are Dried Fruits Higher in Sugar Than Fresh?* Verywell Fit. https://www.verywellfit.com/why-are-dried-fruits-higher-in-sugar-than-regular-fruit-2506131

Marengo, K. (2020, February 7). *Refined carbs: What they are, and how to avoid them.* Www.Medicalnewstoday.com. https://www.medicalnewstoday.com/articles/refined-carbs

Martínez Steele, E., Baraldi, L. G., Louzada, M. L. da C., Moubarac, J.-C., Mozaffarian, D., & Monteiro, C. A. (2016). Ultra-processed foods and added sugars in the US diet: evidence from a nationally representative cross-sectional study. *BMJ Open*, *6*(3), e009892. https://doi.org/10.1136/bmjopen-2015-009892

Nguyen, P. K., Lin, S., & Heidenreich, P. (2016). A systematic comparison of sugar content in low-fat vs regular versions of food. *Nutrition & Diabetes*, *6*(1), e193–e193. https://doi.org/10.1038/nutd.2015.43

Rana, S. (2017, December 5). *Fruit Juice Versus Whole Fruit; Which One Should You Choose?* NDTV Food. https://food.ndtv.com/food-drinks/fruit-juice-versus-whole-fruit-which-one-should-you-choose-1781956

Srour, B., Fezeu, L. K., Kesse-Guyot, E., Allès, B., Méjean, C., Andrianasolo, R. M., Chazelas, E., Deschasaux, M., Hercberg, S., Galan, P., Monteiro, C. A., Julia, C., & Touvier, M. (2019). Ultra-processed food intake and risk of cardiovascular disease: prospective cohort study (NutriNet-Santé). *BMJ*, l1451. https://doi.org/10.1136/bmj.l1451

11 No-Sugar Snacks That Skip the Refined Stuff but Not the Flavor. (2018, May 3). Greatist. https://greatist.com/eat/no-sugar-snacks#1

Tarlton, A. (n.d.). 19 Delicious Desserts You'd Never Know Are Sugar-Free. Taste of Home. https://www.tasteofhome.com/collection/deliciou s-sugar-free-desserts/

Printed in Great Britain
by Amazon